# ULTIMATE BODY

## AWESOME ABS!

**Robert Marting, B.S., Exercise Science**

**Disclaimer:** No portion of text in this book may be used or reproduced in any manner whatsoever without expressed written permission except for the use of brief quotations appearing in articles or reviews. The methods and information explained within this book are not medical advice but rather represent the author's opinions and are solely for informational and educational purposes.

Robertmarting.com, its officers or affiliates are not responsible in any manner whatsoever for injury or health condition that may occur through following the programs, food choices or opinions expressed herein. There are inherent risks involved with any exercise or nutritional programming and because of these risks, it is entirely under your own free will and discretion to follow any activity described herein. All nutritional information is presented for informational purposes only and may not be appropriate for all individuals. Consult with your physician and/or qualified dietitian before starting any exercise program or altering your dietary intake to be sure.

Trademark 2018
ISBN 978-0-692-17478-4
www.robertmarting.com

# TABLE OF CONTENTS

# Acknowledgements

There are a few professional colleagues and friends I would like to sincerely thank for their support and contributions to the completion of this book.

Steven John Smith, DVM of http://www.homepetdoctor.com for his dedication to not only training with me like there is no tomorrow but his patience and persistence in helping finalize this book. He somehow found time to do it while saving our furry friend's lives full-time.

Armando Gutierrez, owner of FFTC https://fitnessandfuncenters.com/ and professional colleague for allowing me to shoot photographs for this book at all hours. Thanks Mondo, you've been a great friend and motivator.

Cory Sorensen http://www.corysorensen.com who took the great cover shot of this book and countless other amazing photographs for me and others in fitness, or anything else for that matter. Thanks for the work and friendship over the years Cory!

# Preface

I would like to thank you for purchasing this book, supplement to the resistance training DVD series *GREAT FORM EQUALS GREAT RESULTS.* I would also like to congratulate you for taking this very important first step in creating a stronger and healthier you. I sincerely value the opportunity to help you reach your goals in fitness and beyond. After all, it's not where you start but where you end up. Just remember what you learn along the way and have fun while you get there!

I wrote this book for a couple of reasons; one being that fitness has been my passion for as long as I can remember. After being in this business now for well over a decade, I must say I am getting really tired of seeing people being taken advantage of by slick marketers selling people bogus supplements, gizmos and empty promises. Our nation is in an epidemic state with adult and childhood obesity at over 60% of the population being overweight and the numbers are climbing with various spin-off conditions of obesity- diabetes, heart disease and cancer just to name the big three. What we need are sound solutions to getting our country back in better shape and health, back to basics so to speak. With that I wanted to put together a collection of real information that works, dispel all the myths out there and convey an easy to understand plan of attack to achieve your best shape ever and make it last. After all it's easy to understand how we got to this point. Our society is one of excess and convenience. I'm all for convenience but not to the point of causing more harm than good! We all deserve to have the body and life of our dreams yet the health and fitness industry has become clouded by so much misinformation and empty promises- all to make a quick buck. It seems more difficult than ever to find or even believe what works and what is a total waste of time or money. Let me just tell you from my experience that it is easier than you think to get there, especially if you apply the correct information. You now have that information at your fingertips!

This book is for you if:

- You're tired of spending your money on empty promises, bad diet books and useless infomercial equipment
- You've tried every liquid, low-carb, low-fat, veggie, cookie-fad diet out there, losing a few pounds at the onset only to gain twice as much back a couple months later (hint- fad diets do not work)
- Week in and week out you hit the gym or attempt to workout without a plan, not seeing much change in your body, if any
- You have tried different exercise "routines" and spent too much money on unqualified trainers, not getting the results you want
- You're ready to finally get the body you want and keep it for the long term
- You want to improve the quality of every aspect of your life
- You're ready to actually see your ABS!
- *You can have the body and life you want.*

I've seen and worked it all. I've done countless magazine spreads, covers, fitness infomercials and promotional work for supplement companies. I can share an insider's view of the fitness industry to help you weed out the garbage and focus on what works. I have to say that some of the products actually do offer some value but most of them don't.

Like many other industries, most products that sound too good to be true probably are. There is no magic pill for getting the body you want, at least for now. We've all seen countless gizmos and supplements that promise you results, but you have to understand the closest thing we have to that magic pill is consistent exercise and smart eating habits. We need to start taking an interest in our own health and fitness. The greedy pharmaceutical companies aren't going to do it for you; the sicker we get, the more dependent we become on their medicines and the more cash they make. But why let ourselves get to that point in the first place? Why not take the position of heading illness off, before it starts?

I don't know about you but I would rather prevent the cause than have to treat the disease. The countless hokey supplement companies sure aren't going to look out for your health either; they just pull the wool over your eyes with claims that their quick fixes can melt fat right off your belly, virtually overnight. They like the fact that people keep getting fatter and fatter; they target this problem and actually profit off of the sense of hopelessness that some people develop about their weight. The solution isn't within a bottle of fat-loss pills or surgery. It's sad to me that every other billboard I see now is advertising the "miracle" fat-loss surgical procedure of the month. I'm aware that it's needed for certain cases, but why go under the knife when all it takes is smart eating habits and effective exercise tactics to avoid an extreme surgery? I'm not talking about walking around the block or mindless tread milling (dread-milling as I call it), I'm talking about smart resistance training at a quick and potent intensity.

Long, boring cardio on a dread-mill? Sure, it's better than nothing but if you want *Ultimate* results I invite you to change the way you look at fitness altogether. Of all the modes of exercise out there, resistance training is the one that can dramatically change the shape of your body and maintain a healthy bodyweight for the long term but you have to do it right. These are tactics for life and not an "extreme" time-limited plan designed to leave you hanging and guessing what to do next after sixty, ninety, or X number of days as some programs practice. Establish your goals, learn the proper methods, become proficient at them and continue to improve for the rest of your life. You will soon become a pro at programming your mind and body for success.

As a professional it is my job to pass along information that is real, that dispels the myths and exposes the garbage out there. I wrote this book to change lives by providing the exact methods to achieve your best body ever, Abs included! It's time to take control of your health and life. **If you don't, who will?**

It's time to make it happen.

# CHAPTER 1: Claim Your Motivation!

## *What's yours?*

Consider why you want to change and consider it often! I wanted to start with this topic because knowing why will help propel you through your workouts, your meal plan and ultimately get you to your best body ever. It may seem basic but it helps to identify what is going to push you through your transformation. Sometimes (myself included) you need everything you can wrap your head around to help elevate your mindset to get through the day or week- or in our case the next session! DON'T forget the reason you want to improve your body and your life!

The reason can be anything. Just refer to it, make a note of it and if it's in photo form, post it somewhere where you can see it regularly. This way, when it's hard to muster up the energy to train you have your #1 reason staring you in the face. Think about it for a minute, identify it and remember it. As a Trainer I love to hear the reasons my clients wish to train and motivate themselves. I would love to hear yours, so email it to me at *email@robertmarting.com* I strive for constant improvement: this means that I never stop learning; some of my clients have taught me much on the subject over the years.

## *Sticking to it!*

### Realize our bodies are made for movement.

This notion may seem like common sense yet it never ceases to amaze me the number of people that still fall into the opposite way of thinking. This is for those people: We were NOT meant to sit in cubicles all day, soak our spines and brains in caffeine while stiffening our joints and shrinking our muscles in the process. Our bodies are anabolic machines, meant to use food (of the healthy type) to fuel our muscles to perform work. Long ago this meant we moved a lot to perform that work, but in today's automated world many of us are forced into roles of inactivity and our health has taken it on the chin- or waistline to be more accurate. Think about it for a second, long ago there was no obesity epidemic, we didn't put all that shelf-life extending, artery-hardening transfat and saturated fat in our food and we moved a lot more. Well, it's time to go back to basics. It's just plain good for us.

Think of how much more productive, happy and capable you'll be when you're in the body you want- you'll be more athletic, happy and healthy. This is our goal. This is what we strive for- to live leaner, stronger and more active.

### Welcome adversity and take it head on.

When you expect difficulties, they don't hit you as hard. Chances are good that you're more prepared and that you have a plan to circumvent them. After all, this is life. People that run from challenges never hit their goals. People that embrace adversity however, have a plan of action and this usually starts with realizing that nobody is immune from adversity. It makes us stronger. I thank my father for saying to me "Welcome to real- world 101" He was right. Life is full of challenge and sacrifice. Anyone who states the contrary is selling something. The take-home message from this is the *growth* that can result from these challenges!  Physically and emotionally. Just know that life is going to throw things at us, try to trip us up and take the wind out of our sails; it's normal. Turn those hurdles into positive energy and use them to improve. Training for ultimate results is a great classroom for this!

## Take an attitude of gratitude.

This book is about basic methods that work and this topic is no different. For me, when I feel like I can't get out of bed or am thinking about using some weak excuse not to workout, I think of all of the people in the world that wish they could do just that. Some would kill to be able to get out of the wheelchair or bed they are confined to and simply walk. The take home lesson: health is the true wealth. This can be applied across the board as well. I use it when I'm having a less-than-positive type of day.  Just remember if you have your health, you have wealth and the problems we face all of the sudden aren't worth stressing over.

## Be attentive to what you want.

Fact: We bring more of whatever it is we focus on the most to fruition; our energy will target what our attention is on.  Where are you focusing your energy? Is this thing what you want more of? If it's achieving the best shape of your life then stay focused on that thought, nonstop. When you are presented with a thought that could sway your focus off of the desired path ask yourself "Is this going to help me reach my goal?"

## Focus on constant improvement.

No matter how small or seemingly insignificant, because that's not the case. Any improvement on any scale is one worth celebrating because you are moving closer to you goal and staying on course to achieve it. Don't focus on reaching perfection. The ultimate challenge of life is not a race to the finish but an evolving quest to become better. Improvements in realistic smaller increments translate to less of a chance you will falter and give up. This builds confidence and proves you can do it. Progression is victory.

## The time is NOW- and it's a daily commitment.

Choosing to make a positive change in your life is an "in the moment" gut check. You have to ask yourself (and be honest) "In this space in time do I want to remain the same old me or do I want to make a step toward the person I know I can be?" Make the choice and remind yourself why the old you just won't cut it anymore. Your results await!

## If it's not going to support your efforts, delete it.

This can be anything in your life that is not going to help you advance to your main goal of an amazing body and a great set of ABS, but mainly I'm referring to people. Sometimes these "negateurs" that pose as friends to us can hold us back, bring us down and ultimately impede us from achieving our goals. Why? Simple. Misery loves company and some people just can't handle the thought of being outshined. Get rid of them. Maybe give them one chance to be positive and support you. The second they say anything like "you can't" or question your choice in a negative manner it's time to show them the door. You could try to put on the kid gloves and tell them you want to improve your life on all fronts and you would like them to do it with you- then see what they say. It's your call, but in my experience if these types of "friends" (or even family) won't support something as positive as this in your life then it's time to cut the dead weight and hope the best for them (can you tell I've faced some resistance to my fitness endeavors myself?) You can't save anyone from themselves, and it's best to hang with people that will INSPIRE you to be your best and not keep you from it.

## Be kind to yourself, be forgiving.

Ok, so you're on the program and nothing is going to stop you from getting the body you want. There's no better way to set the standard for yourself than that. All I want to say here is this: you will trip up, you will miss workouts and you will have more than one "cheat day" with food in a row. If not, then I could learn from you! When this happens, don't worry about it. We all have some need of instant gratification inside of us somewhere. The feeling we get after the fact can be one of guilt or shame. Nobody is infallible. Don't beat yourself up; learn from it and find out a little bit more about yourself as you go. Chances are good that you'll find out exactly what your trigger points are each time you're getting off track and eventually you'll know how to handle them.

## Know what you're doing before you hit the gym.

I know, that's why you're reading this book right? How many times have you seen people in any gym over a period of a year, or even two or three years- never change how their body looks? I see countless people in the gym that sort of wander through their workouts, not really having the specific plan mapped out for what they are doing that day. Now, there could be any number of reasons for the lack of progress. Form and intensity are the two most obvious culprits. The other ones are volume and consistency.

For me, at this stage of the game I don't keep a training log but I recommend one for people just starting out. I know just from repetition what muscle group I am working any given day and which exercises to choose. It gets very easy over time to just know what needs to be done, no pen and paper required. You will get there too. The point being you know what you're doing when you step foot in the gym and you have clear-cut goals- to put pure focus on the muscle group or method for that day get the most out of your efforts- no guess work, just progress.

## Get a training partner.

This one can really help in countless ways. It's really great for those just starting out because you and your partner can feed off of each other's energy and positive feedback. Having a spotter there to help push you through your sets is a priceless advantage when it comes to results too. But for me (yes, even I have challenges staying motivated) when a buddy is waiting for me or on the way to train with me, I know I have to go. It's not a good feeling to stand anyone up. If you have trouble finding a training partner, email me. I will be a stand-in training partner with you online- email@robertmarting.com

## Visualize your ULTIMATE body and life you want to create.

Now take the steps to get there. This is such a powerful tool and to not mention it would be a disservice. This principle can be applied to every aspect of your life. Before you take on anything that could be challenging, stop for a moment and rehearse in your mind how you want it to turn out. For example, a new workout or lift you'll learn from me in this book. Visualize yourself making it happen with perfect and intense form to evoke the best possible result. Now take it a step further and visualize the life you wish to be living. Do this every day and soon you won't be visualizing it, you'll be living it. A skinny kid in rural Texas, I used this technique for years and the pictures in my mind ended up on the covers of magazines.

## Allow me to help you succeed.

I know what it's like to abandon your goals and it's not fun. For whatever reason, if you are thinking about quitting or don't feel you have the energy to continue on, please contact me. You're not alone on this journey- don't throw in the towel. Feel free to contact me with any questions or issues you may have with making the choice to change, nutritional or training issues at www.robertmarting.com -my official blog site. Assistance is just an email away and I will hold myself to doing whatever I can to help keep you on track.

## *My take on Trainers*

Fitness is empowering. Not just from the physical benefits but more importantly what it can do for our mindset- every aspect of our lives can be enhanced. As a fitness professional, I'm just as much an educator as I am a motivator. Some people need that regular in-your-face motivation from their trainers, especially in the beginning. The monetary incentive and just the pure fact that someone is waiting for you at the gym or coming to your house makes it easier to commit. Those things are great, indeed.

In my opinion, the best trainers articulate their knowledge in such a way that the client will understand how to apply it themselves and how to use it for life, in their own unique way. I don't think the ultimate goal of a trainer should be to keep coming back for more sessions or for the client become dependent on them. When the client is self-sufficient, up to speed and motivated to strive for constant improvement, they don't really need a trainer anymore. That is ultimate success in my mind. They can apply the tools I present to them for life, expand on them, grow and reach their ultimate potential. This is what a separates a good trainer from a great trainer- that's just my take.

# CHAPTER 2: Why Weight Training?

Easy answer. Lift weights to lose weight! (more importantly, to lose inches) Our bodies are machines so to speak, using mechanical advantages to perform work. Our joints and the muscles that flex and extend them must be maintained to stay in top working order and help hinder the development of arthritic conditions. The same maintenance is given to the cars we drive so why not our bodies? Of all the different modes of exercise out there, weight training is the one that can turn your body into an around-the-clock fat burning furnace. We are talking overall fat and stored energy expenditure here. More muscle on your body as a whole does the most damage to fat stores. Don't worry, I'm not going to bore you with the physiology of how this is possible but it will benefit you to know some basics and understand what's going on inside your body.

Muscle and fat are archenemies. You've probably heard that muscle weighs more than fat; that's sort of a misstatement. If you put a pound of muscle and a pound of fat side by side, each one stills weighs a pound, but they occupy different volumes of space. Muscle is about 18% more dense than fat. The pound of muscle would be roughly the size of a baseball; the pound of fat would be three times the size of the muscle and look like a squiggly mass of cloudy, yellow Jell-O. Pretty disgusting, but remember that visual! You can see by this example that you could actually lose inches off your waist but remain around the same weight. This is why it's important to use a tape measure to track your progress and not so much a scale. When your clothes start fitting more loosely you will know what I'm talking about!

For the novice, improvement will be noticed relatively quickly in the beginning, with noticeable results in the first one to three months. This is normal, as your body is basically in shock and quickly deals with the new stresses you are putting on it. As time passes, muscle gains (and body fat loss) will arrive more slowly as your body adapts. We can combat this with drastic changes in our training regimen; it keeps your body guessing and pushes more results. No two workouts are ever the same for me- the body responds and adapts very well to routine stress so we will continue to challenge it with different angles, order of exercise and weight or rep schemes. In other words, don't let your routine become routine! This will confuse it into improving even more. We may use the same exercises, but we'll shift around the order, increase the weight, use different techniques like drop-sets and supersets to switch it up often. This is coined the "muscle confusion" principle and it has been around for decades.

And then the real magic starts: the afterburn. This means that muscle increases your metabolism long after you are finished lifting weights. Does this mean the more muscle you have the more fat you will burn? Absolutely. How about while at rest or even sleep? Yep, weight training has us covered there too. Exercise scientists call this effect

EPOC, an acronym for Excess Post-exercise Oxygen Consumption. This boils down to how fuel is used preferentially, hinging upon how your body stores are maintained. We're going to touch on this in chapter 6. But for now, take a quick look at this chart. Muscle is an active tissue: each pound of new muscle you put on your body will burn about 60 calories per day. This can really add up and slim you down.

| Pounds of New Muscle | Pounds of fat burned per month | Pounds of fat burned per year |
|---|---|---|
| 1 | 0.5 | 6 |
| 3 | 1.5 | 19 |
| 5 | 2.6 | 31 |
| 10 | 5.1 | 62 |
| 12 | 6.2 | 74 |
| 15 | 7.7 | 93 |
| 20 | 10.3 | 123 |

Amazing? You bet. It's easy to see how weight training can get you the body and ABS of your dreams when you see numbers like that. You can and will get the results you want!

OK, but what kind of weight training? What types of lifts? In what order? Which exercises? I'm going to cover each specific exercise in the following chapters. Then, I'm going to show you how to construct the best order of exercises for your body type and goals in mind.

After training vigorously with some good intensity, your blood and muscle glucose levels will be much lower than when you started. Low glucose levels signal the body to preferentially burn fat; the body switches into that mode that after intense training, and more muscle makes this possible.

Muscle burns fat! Period! I got myself into cover-model shape from smart eating and a powerful combination of weight-training workouts. Not from AB gizmos or endless cardio. As a matter of FACT, I can count the times I have been on a treadmill on ONE hand the past five years and those times were for a magazine shoot. That's not saying I don't head outside and sprint a few hills now and then- it's more effective and builds fat-burning muscle. My cardio-respiratory system gets a real workout as well and in less time than any treadmill could offer. Your body is the machine!

Too much attention has been given to dieting or cardio alone and not enough attention to weight training. Let's quickly go over some of the main reasons weight training is a must-have in the quest for the Ultimate Body:

In addition to the fore-mentioned, strong muscles are great for your heart. This is because they are able to perform better with less oxygen, meaning the heart doesn't have to pump as hard when you are active. Safe to deduct that strong muscles are good for your blood pressure.

Lifting weights protects your joints and back. Not only do your muscles get stronger, so do the connective tissues. You put less stress on them because the muscle tissue can take on greater workloads- awfully important for preventing and treating arthritis. Just make certain you use GREAT FORM. When you train with proper form in the correct biomechanical pathways you strengthen your joints very effectively.

Weight training drastically improves your looks. Lean muscle tissue is taut against your body, as opposed to fat or flab, which jiggles and sags.

Weight training gives you a mental boost. You just feel stronger and are able to take on everyday tasks much easier and this does wonders for your mind and outlook. Others will take notice.

Weight training requires active living. As I mentioned at the onset, there are no magic pills, foods or secret supplements that give you a strong, lean body. Only weight training correctly can achieve this. Nothing depletes your health worse than sedentary living and the fact you have strength training on your side is an actual true "secret" weapon.

## *Myths dispelled!*

After too much time now I am happy to report that the consensus is increasing, weight training can benefit everyone and is finally getting the respect it deserves. Even the medical community is now recommending that all adults train their major muscle groups at least once a week. (Although many MD's I know could also benefit from a solid training and nutrition plan.) Let's set the record straight here and talk about myths or misconceptions about nutrition and weight training. I can't tell you how many times I have heard these from various clients or people in gyms all over the world.

### It doesn't matter which you do first, cardio or weights.

If you want to build and keep fat-burning muscle it sure does. The reason is simple; Glycogen. All that fresh, stored energy needs to be used for an all-out effort in the weight room. What you need to remember here is that the way you will perform the weight training will be cardio in its own right. Many times I have felt like I have just ran a 400 meter sprint after a great session with weights. And the metabolic benefits of a weight training program are far more powerful than a cardio program alone. Save the cardio until after your training session with weights. Very rarely do I do sprints and weights on the same day. Pressed for time or if I missed a session here and there I go hit the hill sprints in the morning and then mid afternoon I'm on the weights. It works for me, but I know some people don't have that kind of time and I avoid it too if I can. Look, both modes of training are intense. That's what it's about. Don't overdo it especially once you know how to tap into intensity. The motto is simple here: build muscle, burn fat around the clock.

## "Low carb" diets are a realistic way to lose weight

Nope. That's a fad term and diet. I just refer to it as the "smart carb" diet. You can actually lose weight for the very short term, but that's only because of water and salt weight. For every one gram of carbohydrate, there are three grams of water. So, if you get on some carb-restricted diet, sure you'll lose some fast weight but it's usually muscle and water loss. Fat is what we want gone forever and low carb diets don't deliver long term. The pounds end up coming back and usually more than before you started the low carb diet. It's just not a realistic weight management solution. We need carbs for energy. Just make sure you get them from the smart sources (listed in Chapter 5) those will help you lose fat through insulin release management. These carbs will feed fat burning muscle, starve fat cells and do it long-term.

## You must follow the same "routine"

You may have heard this from different fitness companies as of late, some call it the "muscle confusion" principle. It has actually been around a long time and it just refers to not letting the muscles get used to the same routine to stay stimulated, challenged and growing.

It's actually an old bodybuilding term from back in the day, it's just being renamed by a few companies trying to take credit. The reason it has been around so long is that it works and I've been practicing it for years. For me (as it will be for you) no two workouts are the same. I use the same movements but I perform them using different weights and sequences each time I train- but always intensity. Coin it whatever you want, muscle confusion or training trickery. It's all the same so mix up each workout. That way, the muscles never get used to the same series of movements. I still start with a compound movement because that way I can recruit the most muscle fibers and release more fat-burning HGH. I just pick a different compound movement than I did the previous workout. You know how routine gets boring for us? The same thing day in, day out? Our muscles react in the same exact way. This isn't good for the amazing body we are trying to build. Keep them guessing and interested, your mind will also benefit from mixing it up often!

## Sit-ups and crunches are the best way to lose belly fat and see your Abs.

This has got to be one of the biggest misunderstandings in the fitness world. The actual fact of the matter (or many facts) is that the opposite is true. You read that right, you don't have to do any of those exercises to have your Abs show up.  Mind you, your Abs are a muscle group and must be trained and rested just as any other group like chest or back. The difference is this: We all have abdominal muscles- we all should come into this world with all the same muscles for that matter; some of us have more developed Abs than others, but Abs we all have. They are usually just covered up by a layer of belly fat. We have to remove this layer of fat to see them. Simple as that. We do this by smart eating habits and proper training methods you have within these pages. Of all my years of getting my Abs on the covers of major fitness magazines, the mainstay of getting that lean was performing fat-burning compound movements with supersets, supplemented with some abdominal movements. This again is where the beauty of effective weight training comes in. When you build more muscle strategically around your body, that muscle is going to act as a fat-burning furnace than never shuts down. As long as you're alive and as long as you maintain habits to support that muscle, it will continue to be fat's enemy number one and will burn it up appropriately. Keep reading!

## You should eat one gram of protein per pound of bodyweight.

Maybe, but that's probably too much. Your body will store that extra protein as fat. A more realistic and safer way to start would be to take in 1-1.5 grams of protein per pound of lean body mass- which is what your body weighs minus the fat: your muscles, bones and organs. To calculate it easily, use the following example: If my body weight is 200 lbs and my body fat is measured at 25%, then I would simply multiply 200 x .25 equaling 50 which gives me my body fat in pounds. I then subtract 50 from 200. This gives me 150 pounds of lean body mass. As a side note using body fat calipers to measure your body fat percentage is one of the more reliable methods to use. Just make sure you get measured by someone who is trained well in the practice and go with the average. It's never a single number but a range.

To sum it up, if your total body weight is 200 pounds, and your body fat percentage is 25%:

- 200 x .25 = 50 lb of body fat from 200lbs = 150lbs of lean body mass.

## You can have "sculpted" or "longer" muscles.

Ok. Right. Does your training gizmo or secret include free bone-lengthening surgery as well? You don't get longer muscles, ever. Leaner is a more believable description. Our muscles are attached to bones and they don't lengthen beyond those insertion and origin points. This is entirely dependent upon one thing: genetics. Now, once you properly fuel your body with the right nutrients and correctly challenge it to build more muscle will it appear to have "longer" or "leaner" muscles- we simply utilize effective methods to achieve that look. And yes, this look can help you "appear" taller as well. The "toned" or "sculpted" buzz words offer the same soft language meant to sell some silly contraption. Our muscles don't know sculpting and they don't know toning, all they know is resistance and the capacity to perform work. Let them appear "sculpted" by increasing the fiber count and stripping off the layer of subcutaneous body fat!

## Muscle turns to fat as you get older.

This couldn't be more incorrect. Muscle and fat are two totally different tissues. What actually happens is that over time if someone fails for whatever reason to maintain the workout schedule they have been performing the muscle actually will shrink. Not always the case but it is safe to say this person might be eating higher calorie, fattier foods as well, so their body fat may increase at the same time. Due to these changes in habit it's understandable how one could think muscle just "turns" into fat. In order for muscle to remain we have to train it consistently. If we don't, it will shrink in size or atrophy. Fat cells on the other hand just increase in size if we feed them and remain sedentary so they end up covering the shrinking muscle tissue. Fat is not a very metabolically active tissue. Feed the muscle, starve the fat and TRAIN! Again, muscle eats up fat around the clock! Remember this when you're burning through your supersets! (more on this later)

## Woman get large, bulky muscles if they lift weights.

Again, this is another big misconception. Most men can't even get the muscle size they want let alone women and they have the testosterone to do it! This result requires a type of lifting and intensity that most of us just don't need to perform. The other element needed for large bulky muscles is the fact you have to eat an incredible amount of calories to do this. Unless you're a linebacker in the NFL, I wouldn't worry about that kind of intake, it's just not practical. Further, women just don't have the hormones needed for bulky muscle growth. Now, there are always exceptions. Some people are gifted with fast-twitch fibers for explosive power and capacity for larger muscles (like sprinters) as opposed to slow twitch (distance runner types) but those people are pretty rare. Most woman who practice correct weight training techniques will lose inches, start seeing their Abs, achieve shape and curves they want, become better athletes and lose a few pounds to boot especially if they smartly reduce their caloric intake. The point to drive home out of this is that the average woman can elicit an HGH response through proper weight lifting and burn fat from it. One pound of fat and one pound of muscle still weigh the same, only that one pound of fat takes up 5 times the space as the one pound of muscle. So which would you rather have on your frame? Me too.

## Weight training makes you slow, stiff and inflexible.

False. Again, this is what GREAT FORM is all about! There is this thing called full range of motion (ROM), which means that any given movement brings a joint throughout its full capacity of movement from full flexion to full extension. When the joint is fully extended, you are in essence stretching the muscle while at the same time strengthening it. I'm not saying you should abandon your stretching routine but when performed properly weight training can lengthen and stretch the muscles very effectively. How many "slow" sprinters do you see? Right. Not many, not ever. Why? Because they lift weights and they nurture the fast-twitch fibers they have to be leaner, lighter and more explosive off the blocks. Sprinters arguably have the best physiques on the planet and they train with weights.

## I'm too old to start lifting weights.

This is blatantly false and sadly a product of our society. In various exercise science studies, people in their seventies and eighties began a weight training regimen and showed significant gains in muscle growth and strength. They were able to take on day-to-day tasks much more easily, and the training even helped to better protect them against falls. Some of the participants could scarcely walk at the beginning of the program and could walk much easier after training for just a few weeks. Amazing! In another study, it was shown that weight training can actually slow or stop the aging process in our muscles! No matter what society has led us to believe, the true fact of the matter is you don't have to grow out of shape as you age and quite the opposite is true: You can improve at any age!

## Some exercises "shape" the muscle and some "build mass".

It's not the movement that dictates the type of muscle adaption, but the INTENSITY and number of repetitions performed. Weight training routines and goals are totally scalable just like any other type of training. Now, certain compound movements like the bench press or squat are better for the quest for mass because you have the help of two or more muscles helping to move more weight, which is better for higher intensity sessions and HGH release. It is these same movements in fact that will make you leaner and help expose your Abs as well. But if I did lighter, less intense bench presses and then did heavier, more intense cable flies I would prompt more growth from the flies. Muscles don't know shaping or mass. They only respond to intense workloads and are forced to grow from stress. Don't forget about consuming the necessary calories to get "big"- which takes dedication all by itself. The fact of the matter here is that most people (men included) find it extremely challenging to get that bulky look. Some do want that and it is totally achievable. You just have to train for the desired result that you want. As you'll soon find out, training with a set of specific methods geared for lean muscle growth and increased heart rate will chisel a rock-hard body and set of Abs like you never dreamed.

## "Core stability" exercises are the best way to get a ripped set of Abs.

Guess what? Wrong again. This is another fad term that is being tossed around by too many novice trainers in the fitness industry. If you've been in any of these large-chain gyms in past few years you've seen what I'm talking about: Some random trainer balancing their client on a stability ball or balance board while at the same time making them do a set of bicep curls. They try to sell you on the fact that you're about to fall over (and twist an ankle or sprain a knee) activates your "core" and gives you ripped Abs! When you learn how and what type of weight training movements to perform you automatically engage your "core." Further, these same movements will systematically put more lean muscle on your frame, which will burn the fat off of your body like a hot knife through butter.

## *Terms and methods to apply*

Let's start with one of the more basic yet most important concepts when it comes to results, INTENSITY. How much effort you put into each workout, each set, down to each rep. To be more clear, the definition explains it as an extreme degree of strength, force, energy or feeling.

Ok, let's apply this to any given workout, down to each set and repetition. I want you to be totally focused on the task at hand. To be able to feel the muscle being challenged, you have to put effort into the work being performed. Another way to put this is if your friend was trying to talk to you during your set, you would be too into the zone and you wouldn't really notice them. Focus. Mindset. This is what it is all about. Get intense, get results. Fast. You don't know how many times I have come across people in the gym, even many "Trainers" that do not apply this most basic rule of results to their client's or even their own workouts for that matter. In terms of an intense set an easy way to measure intensity is towards the end of the set. When you have the right weight selected and you are working on completing a set of 8 or so reps, it should be difficult for you to complete number 6, 7 and almost impossible to complete number 8. This is intensity at work. I cringe when I see people in the gym carrying on a conversation during their "weight lifting" workouts; usually single arm bicep curls. These are the same people that complain about how weight training does nothing for them.

**REPETITION (rep)-** The number of times you do anything, in this case times you perform a proper weight training movement.

**SET-** The group of reps of any given movement. As in: a set of 10 reps of squats.

**AEROBIC-** This refers to an oxygen requirement for exercise, much like a low intensity activity like jogging or easy cycling. Lifting weights is not aerobic. By the time you finish this book you will have a different understanding of aerobic training and what it doesn't do for you.

**ANAEROBIC-** This is what I'm talking about! This means "without oxygen" This type of metabolism occurs during intense physical movements like sprinting or weight training for maximum results.

**MIND-MUSCLE CONNECTION-** This term goes hand in hand with intensity. When you have your mind into the set you can really focus on the feel of each repetition and concentrate on that one thing- feeling the muscle being properly worked, through its full range of motion. When you feel it, you are doing it right with intensity and proper form- the two BIGGEST ingredients to great results in record time. When you're not feeling it, you can probably amp it up a bit and challenge yourself. This is also a good way to stay in tune with your body when it comes to aches and pains that happen for all of us. Listen to your body in and out of the gym but for ultimate results it's a must-have.

**RANGE OF MOTION (ROM)-** Any given joint of the human body has a range of motion. This refers to the full path from full flexion to full extension for any movement. If you don't give your muscles full range of motion, you are cheating yourself out of results. I see it all the time- people using poor form or half reps. Some of the common ones are bench press not going down all the way and tapping the bar on the chest or bicep curls not extending the arms fully at the bottom of the movement. Full ROM is another key ingredient to ensure awesome results. Make sure you use it.

**CONCENTRIC-** This is the phase of a movement that is the "push" and involves the flexing or shortening of the muscle. Conversely for back or pulling movements, the concentric phase would be the pull portion of the lat pull-down. Pushing the weight back up from your chest on a bench press is an example of the concentric part of any given movement. Additionally an important point to make here is that muscle gains in strength, size or power are not made during this phase. Let's talk about where the gains are made in the next term.

**ECCENTRIC-** The phase of the movement where the muscle lengthens and actually produces gains in strength and/or size (also called the negative). On the bench press this is the lowering of the bar to the chest or letting the bar back up during a lat pull-down. When done properly, this is the part of the movement that allows correct full range of motion (ROM) for the best possible results! How many times have you seen people doing half-reps? You are only cheating yourself and not getting the full return on your time invested in training if you don't use this method consistently.

**BREATHING-** Since we're talking about the phases of the movement there is no better time to mention how to breathe during your reps. Inhale on the eccentric and exhale on the concentric. This is especially important if you are pushing a lot of weight but applies for everyone! The more oxygen-rich blood you have being pumped into your muscles, the easier it will be to push or pull it back to the starting position. Breathe and breathe correctly for the best results!

**TEMPO-** I myself like to use an upbeat tempo when I lift. Why? Because it gets my heart beating at a much faster cardio rate. My weight training sessions are more like a sprint than a long-drawn out session of "super-slow" repetitions. For safety's sake it's more important go slower and control momentum during the ECCENTRIC phase of the movement. The CONCENTRIC phase of the movement is usually the faster of the two and can be explained by the ratio 3:1:1- three seconds to lower the weight, one second pause, one second back up to the starting position. I probably use closer to a 2:1:1 and depending on how heavy I'm going, I may not pause at all. The one thing I Absolutely do every time however is a slower controlled eccentric phase for results and safety. The key here is going fast enough to get a good rush of blood into the muscles being trained but being in total control and to not break form. I use a balanced machine-like rhythm until near failure for each set. This ensures I'm challenging my muscles to the point of forcing them to adapt. This gets results. Another way I could explain this is by using the sprinter's physique vs. the long distance runner's physique. If you put these two side by side, who has a more lean, powerful and muscular body? Right, the sprinter hands down. When you train with quick, controlled rep tempo you stimulate your fast-twitch fibers and those are the ones that are wired for muscular growth, speed and power. These all translate to a lean body and of course this leads to Abs!

**COMPOUND MOVEMENT- (CM's)** These are exercises that use more than one muscle or joint that work together to perform, such as the squat or dead-lift. These are far more effective for fat loss and calorie burning. Why? Because you can employ more effort with them thus they set up your body to burn the most calories and fat. Compound movements allow you to use more weight and build more muscle. They are best performed at the START of your weight training session because you need to have that energy readily available to optimally perform the movement and get the most out of it. CM's release more

HGH (human growth hormone) and thus are extremely effective in setting up the body to burn more fat! And by now we know what that means: seeing your Abs!

**ISOLATION MOVEMENT- (IM's)** Simply put, these are movements that use one muscle or joint to perform, like standing bicep curls or tricep pushdowns. These are great movements, but they are refining movements. They don't do much for total functionality, and they don't burn calories as effectively as compound movements. Unless you are using these movements in a superset, save them for the end of your training session. They require less energy to perform and they're great for focusing on a lagging body part or muscle group.

**ATROPHY-** This is what we want to avoid! Greek in origin, it means "ill-fed." It is the wasting away of tissue in the body. In our case this is the breaking down of muscle tissue. We can avoid this by proper weight training and nutrition methods. It is a natural occurrence over time for our muscles to atrophy. Thankfully we can reverse this! Interestingly, astronauts experience major cases of muscle atrophy due to zero-gravity conditions.

**HYPERTROPHY-** Growth! This is what we strive for! Simply put, it is the increase in the volume of an organ or tissue due to the enlargement of its component cells. The most common and visible forms of hypertrophy in skeletal muscle occur as a response to correct weight training techniques- just like the ones you're about to learn. You can increase the rate of muscle hypertrophy with your nutritional intake as well. Just remember that hypertrophy will put your fat burning capabilities into hyper-drive!

**SUPERSET-** This is one of my all-time favorites when it comes to training techniques. It involves performing two exercises back-to-back and combining them into one non-stop set. For example, in one of my informative YouTube videos I superset a home chest workout by combining a set of pushups with a set of free-weight flies. Supersets can be any two movements; I usually perform them in two ways depending upon where I'm training and what is available to me. Most of the time, I will use a push-pull superset scheme: I'll do a pushing movement such as a bench press and then superset it with a pulling movement like a set of bicep curls. So in that case, it's also a compound movement to an isolation movement superset. If you're at home, or in a gym with not much equipment or weight to use, then it makes sense to superset the same muscle group to mimic the effect of heavier weight. Your muscles won't know the difference. All they know is exhaustion. An example of this would be diamond pushups with over-head triceps extensions with a dumbbell. This is an ultra-effective method of weight training as it challenges you to stay focused and complete the set at a machine-like pace; it's what makes lifting weights more of a cardio sprint than a distance race.

**PYRAMID-** This term simply means to increase the weight as you progress with your sets. For example, set one of bicep curls you'll do 30 lbs. for ten reps. Set two, you'll do 40 lbs. and try for ten reps. Set three you'll do 50 lbs. for 8 reps, and so on. It's a very simple tactic but it works like a charm. Why? Because it is progressive resistance and it forces the body to take on more of a workload and adapt much more effectively. It is a way to constantly challenge yourself to improve, and it's also a great mind trick. Progression fuels our minds to perform better. This tactic will push your body to go beyond its comfort zone and give it no choice but to smash through plateaus. Pyramiding your sets is actually a safer way to progress and add weight as well. If you add a little each set, you are essentially preparing your muscles to safely take on more work; this will fine-tune your mind-muscle connection to how certain weights and rep ranges should feel.

A typical pyramid rep scheme on dumbbell bench press for me goes like this:

Set 1- Warm up with 60 lbs, around 20-25 (I usually don't count this as a real set)
Set 2- 15 reps at 75 lbs.
Set 3- 12 reps at 80 lbs.
Set 4- 10 reps at 85 lbs.
Set 5- 8 reps at 90 lbs.
Set 6- 4-6 reps at 95-100 lbs.

If I'm feeling up to it, I will then do a seventh, drop set (see next term) back down to 75 lbs to failure. Pyramiding your sets is a sure-fire way to increase intensity EACH SET. Remember intensity? I will say it again: Intensity with your workouts will give you the intense results you want. Pyramid sets are a great way to continue to get stronger too. You do this by starting your first set with just a little more weight every few workouts.  For example in the scheme above, in a couple weeks I would begin my first real set (set 2) with 80 lbs. instead of the previous 75 lbs. used- thus every set will be increased. This way you are constantly challenging your muscles with more workloads, forcing them to become stronger and capable of increased fat consumption. You won't get as many reps at the onset of each increase, that's normal and just keep pushing. Your body will adapt and you will make great gains in lean muscle and your fat loss will continue to sky-rocket.

**DROP/STRIP SET-** An effective technique and a way to switch it up. Pyramid up to a certain weight, perhaps the heaviest and last set, then work back down to the starting point weight in one painful but result-achieving set. Example: Bicep curls- after that final set of 100 lbs. barbell curls, rack the weight and immediately drop back down to the starting set weight. The result is an amazing pump you won't get from a regular set. It confuses and forces the muscles to work and adapt. The whole idea here is intensity. Can't get away from it can you? Be prepared, this type of training sets your muscles on fire! It's very intense and shouldn't be used that often.

**VOLUME-** The amount of work you perform during each workout. The basic formula for this is Sets x Reps x Weight. For example, in a chest session you lifted 75lbs x 5 reps x 3 sets your total volume would be 1,125lbs. Sounds like a lot of weight and work right? It's actually an example of a low-volume session and wouldn't get you the results you're looking for. Now if you did the same movement but used 60lbs x 12 reps x 3 sets your total volume would be 2,160. To me, volume is just another method to measure intensity or time under tension-the actual time your muscles spend working. Higher volume training is what is needed for hypertrophy. That word can be misleading for some folks in that they don't know that high volume training is most effective for leaning down, burning fat, seeing your Abs and losing inches.

Note that I said inches and not weight. I'm a proponent of high volume training, but I prefer to do it instinctively and I've become quite successful at it. How do I do it? I listen to my body through rep ranges and I use pyramids. By now you know what that means and you can bet it is a way to combine high and low volume modes of training. This bypasses the need to over-think your training sessions. Listen to your body! You'll know if you're not working hard enough; you will for sure after reading this ebook!

**REST AND RECOVERY-** This is a huge determining factor in not only the results you will see for your efforts but also the way you feel and perform overall, in everyday life. All that pushing, pulling, sprinting and sweating are all perceived as one thing to the body: stress. Weight training causes microscopic tears in the muscle fibers; the body protects itself from this stress by building the fibers back stronger and in greater numbers to prepare for more "battle" so to speak. So, adequate rest and recovery time are an absolute must. To build the muscle fibers back up optimally and as fast as possible, it's imperative you get quality rest each and every night. As a matter of fact, gains in muscular strength and/or metabolizing of fat are made when we are at rest, not during the act of training. Specifically, the better the sleep quality you give yourself, the better your results are going to be. REM (rapid eye movement) produces the best HGH (human growth hormone) release and this is what we need for optimal recovery. This usually happens during REM sleep, or when we dream. Depending upon how much intensity you employ and what type of workouts you are enduring, the body should be given at least forty-eight to seventy-two hours before hitting the same muscle group again. If you don't give it the time it needs to repair the stress damage, you will feel it: Not only will you risk injury, you will feel week and not be able to keep challenging yourself higher intensity which will just lead to stalled gains. In my field this is called over-training and it has serious implications like constant fatigue, poor performance at work and the weakening of immune system so colds are more common. I know everyone has their own sleep patterns and requirements (I have to get at least 8 hours per night) but the moral here for the best results, find yours and get the regular rest your body needs. Your training and nutrition must be consistent and your sleeping patterns are no different.

**REST BETWEEN SETS-** This can seriously affect the success or failure of reaching your goals! I'm mainly referring to how much time you should take to rest between sets and this depends mostly on things like your bodytype, type of training and your goals. The rest time between sets will replenish creatine phosphate and/or glycogen which are fuels used for intense anaerobic activity like weight training; somewhere within 30-180 seconds. If you want to get the most out of your training sessions in a short amount of time then try to rest as little as possible between your sets. A great way to ensure this happens is by using **supersets**. On heavier days when I have the inclination to push a lot of weight, I will take more time to recover but across the board this falls in a 45-120 second window. Anything longer than three minutes is too long and just tricks the muscles into thinking that the "battle" is over. Generally, the heavier the weight you use the more rest time is needed between sets. For example, a moderately intense set of eight to twelve reps would require no more than 90 seconds of rest but if you are pyramiding your sets and you perform a tough, heavier set of six to eight reps, then you could rest for up to 2-3 minutes. It all depends on how hard you push yourself and where you are in your session. If at the end, obviously you're going to be a bit more tired and could use more rest time.

**FAST-TWITCH MUSCLE FIBER-** Think Olympic sprinters. Also known as Type II muscle fiber, it has low aerobic power, rapid force development and high anaerobic capacity explosive movements and strength.

**SLOW-TWITCH MUSCLE FIBER-** Think long-distance runners. Also known as Type I fibers, they are generally fatigue-resistant and have a high capacity for aerobic energy supply, but they have limited potential for rapid force development like sprinting.

## *Body Types, Goals and Training*

In the 1940's, American Psychologist William Sheldon came up with the theory of Somatypes. His theory described three basic human body types. Sheldon's work has become a staple in most literature on fitness, nutrition and bodybuilding. Each of the following body types process foods and react to exercise differently, so the type of training, rep/set scheme and focus will depend upon which type you are and your goals. Once you find out which type most suites you and your goals it then becomes much easier to set up your training and nutritional plan for optimum results. Let's dive right in!

## THE ECTOMORPH

Basic characteristics:
- *fragile frame*
- *small-jointed*
- *thin/frail boned*
- *flat-chested*
- *delicate build*
- *usually taller*
- *lightly muscled*
- *large-brained (but not always the wiser)*
- *trouble gaining weight and/or quality muscle*

Picture a distance runner. This is the classic "skinny guy" or "hard gainer" body type. They usually have no trouble eating fatty or high calorie foods and still maintain their skinny look. For most of us, this changes over time due to our metabolism slowing as we age but for some ectomorphs it remains a lifetime challenge to put any quality weight on. That is, if you don't know what you're doing! Most of the people I have encountered that fall under this category make it a goal to add more muscle to their body. After all, there is such a thing as a "skinny-fat body" I'm sure you've seen them- a totally thin body but when they lift up their shirt they have a deposit of excess fat around their belly; this is another example of how over time calories do stack up even for the ectomorphs. So if it's a goal to get more muscle and amp up the metabolism then it's a simple exercise prescription. Ectomorphs need to lift weights and lift rather heavy; using compound movements to release more HGH (human growth hormone). To keep each set and strength levels at an optimum intensity it's beneficial for the ectomorph to take more rest time between sets (90-120 seconds) We can all benefit from having more HGH released and more muscle on our frames, especially as we age. For the ectomorph it can be challenging to put muscle on his/her frame but by no means is it impossible. If this is you, know that you can make great progress. Each body type has the ability to respond to the proper exercise and nutritional plan. I did it and so can you. Plus, your ability to keep fat stores to a minimum is a fortunate thing.

## THE MESOMORPH

Basic characteristics:

- *athletically inclined*
- *leaner, muscular body*
- *medium boned*
- *more mature in appearance*
- *rectangular shape (hourglass for women)*
- *thicker skin*
- *burns fat with relative ease*
- *upright posture*
- *gains or loses weight easily*
- *adds muscle easier and faster*

Picture a sprinter or wrestler. This type has the natural genetics for easy muscle gains and athletic ability- the type that most people loathe because this comes quite naturally to the mesomorph while other body types have to put more work in to get their desired look. Think of an ectomorph's ability to remain thin no matter what they eat and combine that with an easy ability to gain good muscle size quickly. Putting muscle on this type of frame is easy and it's fairly easy to keep fat off as well. A mesomorph has a naturally fit body; maintaining this however still requires a committed schedule of proper training and nutrition just like any other type. Especially as age creeps up, every body type will have to stay on their program to keep improving or maintain the level they like. Meso's get good results from strength training and can use more volume per session than an ectomorph. Just be mindful to not overdo it and listen to your body. Just because you are "gifted" with these genetics does not mean you don't have to work to make progress; maybe just not as hard or in a different fashion but it's work nonetheless!

# THE ENDOMORPH

Basic characteristics:

- *propensity to gain fat*
- *larger boned*
- *soft body*
- *underdeveloped muscles*
- *rounder shaped*
- *over-developed digestive system*
- *difficulty losing weight*
- *usually gains muscle easily*

Picture an offensive lineman or sumo wrestler. An endomorph's strategy should be the loss of excess fat and inches and practicing a lifestyle that keeps them off. This body type must keep a close eye on what they eat; restricting calories (no starvation diets!) and eliminating junk foods, processed foods, sugars and sweets from the diet. Eat frequent and small meals and keep protein intake strong. Use moderate (not heavy) weights at a quick pace while keeping rest between sets to a bare minimum. In addition to the weight training it would be very beneficial to engage in some sort of daily activity like brisk walking or cycling. Swimming is a great choice due to the removal of weight and the pounding that the joints take during other types of activities like running can inflict. If this is your type, you have a good chance of success maximizing your genetics. Just stick to the program, build more muscle, starve the fat and watch the inches and pounds fall off. Many endomorphs have proven it is possible to get great results when you follow the right method!

# CHAPTER 3: The Movements

This chapter is going to cover in text and pictures the same, basic movements I have used over the years, that got my physique (Abs included) on the cover of Men's Fitness magazine. As previously mentioned, muscle loves to burn fat around the clock. You have a choice: you can program your body to store fat, or to burn it in your sleep. When you efficiently build and maintain metabolically active muscle tissue with the techniques shown on these pages, your body will be programmed to keep fat off for the long-term and your "Ultimate Body" will reveal itself!

We're going to start by breaking down each muscle group and describing how to perform each movement in the most efficient and effective way possible. In Chapter 6, we'll take a look at how to put these movements together for complete workout schedules, depending upon your body type and goals. Combining movements creates calorie-scorching supersets for ULTIMATE results. You will learn them all. Another place to see most of these movements is on the DVDs: Great Form Equals Great Results, with the exception of a few new ones!

Remember, we are talking about the most efficient muscle building and calorie burning movements out there, most of which are compound movements (CM's). We'll also cover a few isolation movements for refining your routine or focusing on certain muscle groups, because we all want to improve the small parts as well as the big picture!

## UPPER BODY - CHEST

**PUSH-UP (CM)** The most basic yet effective compound movement for the pushing muscles of the upper body. With all the variations available with push-ups, they allow you to push about 75% of your body weight on average. The Abs are also recruited, as are they are in just about every movement we discuss when done correctly. When we work the Abs without really noticing, that's a beautiful thing. Another benefit of push-ups is that they are easy to vary in terms of angle and intensity. I know you've done push-ups and you know what they look like but let's take a quick look at the proper mechanics of the push-up for ultimate results, as well as some variations to mix it up.

Your body should remain rigid in a straight line from toes touching the ground to top of the head throughout the entire movement. Keep your elbows out relatively wide (but not too wide) from the sides of the body. This places the desired emphasis on the chest. Place your hands in close relation to the sides of the pectoral muscles, approximately two feet apart. Slowly lower yourself to the ground, chest nearly touching the ground and the nose coming close as well with the elbows about 90°.

Press yourself back up to the starting position just short of locking out the elbows. Doing so will keep the desired stress on the chest. If the full version is a challenge, no problem: get a mat or a towel and use your knees as the pivot point. If you want more emphasis on the triceps, bring the hands closer together to form a diamond with the thumb and index finger. It may be beneficial on the wrists to use one of the many push-up grips available these days; I just use a couple of dumbbells as they are just as effective. This makes the movement more challenging because you are able to lower your body a few extra inches and get a better stretch on the pectorals. For even more resistance try propping your feet up on a bench for a decline pushup as seen in the photos.

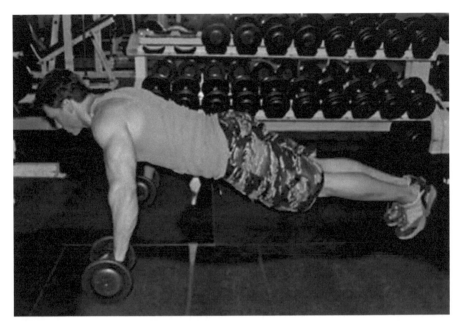

Figure 1: Push up - Starting Position

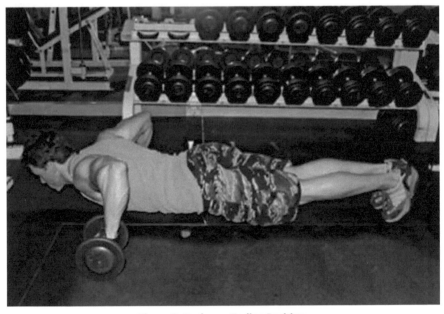

Figure 2: Push up - Ending Position

**DUMBELL PRESS (CM)** This movement is similar to the barbell bench press, except that the longer range of motion inherently possible with dumbbells helps to stretch the pectorals and the extra balance needed with a dumbbell in each hand is also an added challenge to stabilize. To start, have a seat on the bench and place the weights on your thighs. From this position, lean back and slowly use the legs to bring the weights to the starting position. Keep forearms parallel and elbows pulled back. Lower the weights slowly and with control to the stretched position while inhaling a breath.

Press the weights up just short of locking out the elbows and keep the weights at eye level while exhaling. You don't have to touch the weights at the top, just bring them close to each other. Don't "over press" with the shoulders at the top. Allow only the chest to do the pushing. Not locking out your elbows effectively prevents this.

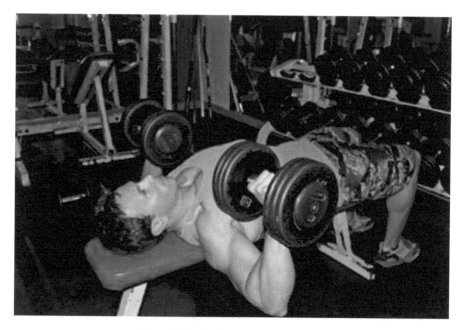

Figure 3: Dumbell Press - Start Position

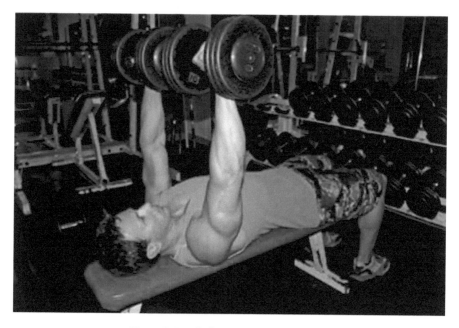

Figure 4: Dumbell Press - Ending Position

**INCLINE FLY (IM)** This movement targets the upper chest directly; the triceps aren't helping push the weight up. For this reason, lighter weights are used (relatively speaking). Begin by placing the weights on each thigh, using the legs to kick them back one at a time into the starting position.

With the arms fully extended and the palms facing one another, lower the weights with the arms perpendicular to the body and elbows pointed to the ground, inhaling a breath. Bend the arms as you lower them, and go as deep as you can to get that comfortable stretch and full range of motion.

Raise the arms back up to the top, as you exhale, returning them to the fully extended starting position. It is an important point to not use too heavy a weight while doing this exercise, as holding the weight further away from the center of your body places extra leverage on the pectorals and the shoulder, so take it easy on this one.

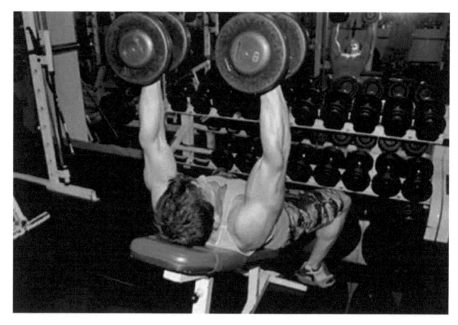
Figure 5: Incline Fly - Start Position

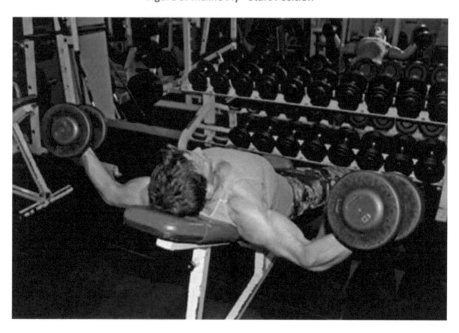
Figure 6: Incline Fly - Ending Position

**INCLINE BARBELL BENCH PRESS (Smith Machine) – (CM)** My favorite compound chest movement. The reasons: it fills in the upper portion of the chest around the top of the sternum (breast bone) and clavicles (collar bones) it builds muscle up top of the chest which over time is pulled down due to gravity. It makes the chest appear thicker and more powerful and that's because it is when you perform this movement correctly.

Men and women alike can benefit from doing incline presses vs. flat presses. Women benefit because, just like for the men (but in a more feminine way) this movement tightens the upper chest area- it pulls things up and keeps them up. I think this is a great reason to do incline presses. This exercise is a great example of how weight training can fight the effects of gravity on our bodies. This one just does the best job!

The execution of this movement is similar to flat barbell bench presses, just incline the bench in the range of 45-50%. We want to keep the emphasis off the shoulders. Some experts advise keeping the elbows in closer to the sides of the body and I think this is a good move; however, I personally put mine out a bit farther. My shoulders handle it well and I feel I get a better stretch on my chest than when I keep them in. Further, it places more stress on my chest. When the elbows are in I feel it a bit more on my triceps and that's not where I want the focus. For the beginners, it's best to keep them in closer. Get the bar off the rack, hold it steady for a second and get your bearings.

SLOWLY bring it down to the top of the chest (two second count) and without bouncing bring it back up. DO NOT jerk the weight back up. Resist the temptation to lock out the elbows, as this makes many beginners put too much shoulder into the top of the movement. You can see this by how they roll their shoulders forward at the top of the movement. If you don't lock out, you avoid this tendency. As with any movement keep a consistent, machine-like pace for the best results. In the photos I am utilizing the versatile Smith press machine to do my incline barbell presses.

41

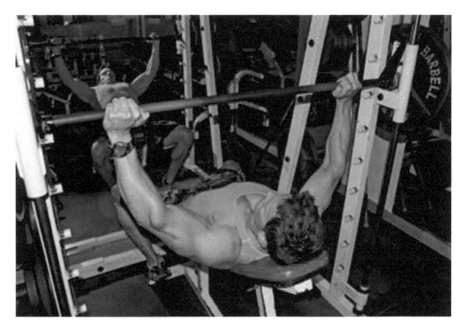

Figure 7: Smith Machine Incline Barbell Press - Starting Position

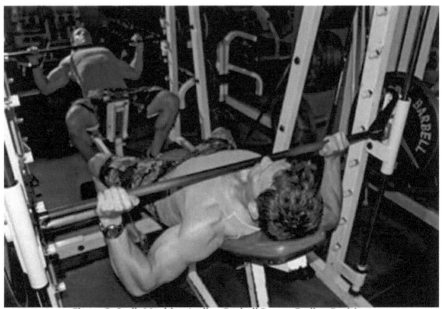

Figure 8: Smih Machine Incline Barbell Press - Ending Position

**SMITH MACHINE BENCH PRESS (CM)** How much can you bench? Forgive me I had to ask. If I made a dime for each time I've been asked that one. Then I see these same people in the gym benching and I fear they're going to rip a shoulder or drop the bar either on their head or crush a sternum.

Let's talk about the movement. Lie on your back on a flat bench. Keep your butt in contact with the bench and your feel flat on the floor. Take an overhand grip on the barbell (for safety and comfort level, wrap the thumb around the bar.) With your hands more than shoulder-with apart, slowly lower the bar to your chest inhaling as you do so, making certain you control the decent of the bar. DON'T bounce the bar off of your chest, but touch it lightly. Exhale as you press the bar back up to the starting position with a hard push. Keep your elbows at your sides to focus on the anterior or front of the shoulders - it's said that this hits the chest more effectively, yet again I prefer to keep mine a bit more outside for a better pectoral stretch.

You can focus of different areas of the chest by lowering the bar to the lower chest for low pec work, mid range for medial pectoral work, or closer to the chin for more upper chest stretch and upper pectoral work. A narrower grip focuses on the inner chest and puts more stress on the triceps; a wider grip focuses on the outer pectorals and takes some stress off the triceps. For me, I keep this one a chest exercise and keep a medium to wide overhand grip. An added note: some prefer to keep their thumb wrapped around the bar; I keep my thumb on the underside of the bar. For beginners I recommend keeping the thumb wrapped for safety.

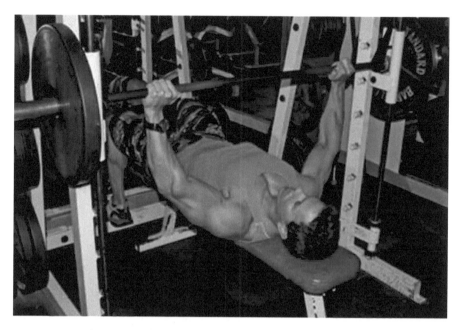

Figure 9: Smith Machine Flat Barbell Press - Starting Position

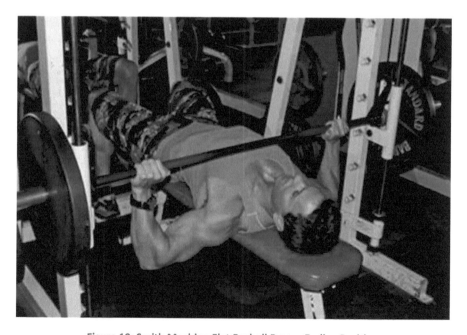

Figure 10: Smith Machine Flat Barbell Press - Ending Position

**INCLINE DUMBELL PRESS  (CM)** Lie back on an incline bench keeping the incline within 45-50 degrees to avoid placing too much emphasis on the shoulders. Begin by placing the weights on your knees and kick the weights back one at a time on each knee to bring them into position. Get your bearings for a second while holding the weights in place above your head.

Slowly lower the weight, keeping the shoulders pulled back moderately and the forearms parallel to each other. Be careful not to let the weights tilt inward towards the body at the bottom of the movement.

I like to pretend I'm holding a bar in my hands this helps me keep the weights straight, and I lose the tendency to tilt them in or out throughout the range of motion. Get a good stretch and come back up to the starting position. Remember your breathing!

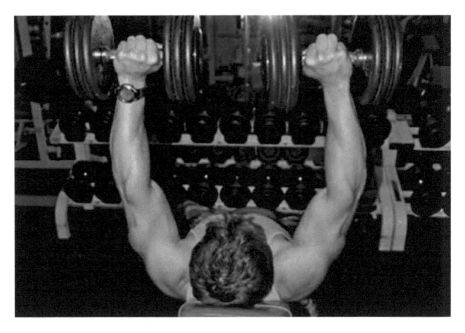

Figure 11: Incline Dumbell Press - Starting Position

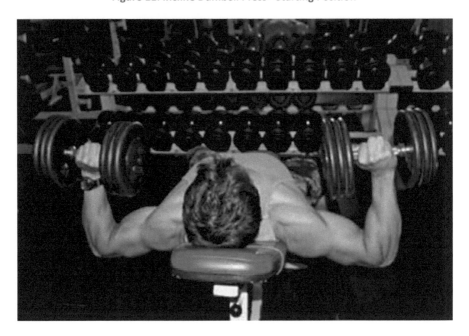

Figure 12: Incline Dumbell Press - Ending Position

**CABLE CROSSOVER FLIES (IM)** This movement mimics the movement of dumbbell flies but makes it harder to cheat. Stand with your feet slightly spread, your body slightly forward, back straight and elbows slightly bent.  Grasp the handles with your arms spread. Inhale and squeeze the cable handles together until they touch, exhaling as you do so and inhaling as your go back to the starting position.

DON'T bend the elbows as you move the cables; the primary joint movement is the shoulders. For this movement strive to keep the elbows locked for the most part. You'll get more out of it by forcing the chest to do most of the work and that's the goal.

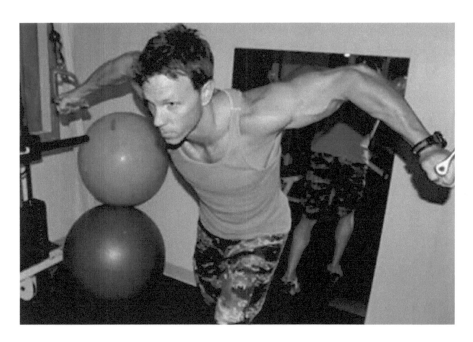

Figure 13: Cable Cross Flies - Starting Position

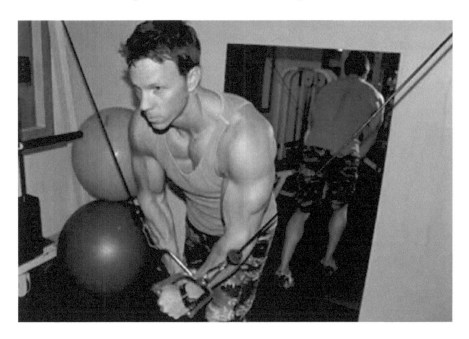

Figure 14: Cable Cross Flies - Ending Position

# UPPER BODY - BICEPS (all movements are IM's)

## STANDING BARBELL BICEP CURL

The standing barbell curl is one of the best if not the best bicep builder of all time. But again it's how intensely and strictly you perform it that gets results.

Begin with your elbows at your sides, arms extended fully to just above touching your thighs with the bar. Slowly curl the bar up not coming up all the way; your forearms should be just under perpendicular to the floor. By doing this you are not letting your biceps rest and this is what we are after combining efficiency with intensity. Slowly lower the bar and repeat reps for a great set.

One topic worth discussing is the cheat or swinging the weight up with momentum. You probably see this as much as I do in the gym. It is not recommended because you may put your back at risk. Although it can be beneficial for growth because you can overload the muscle, which is necessary for growth, I advise using a spotter or strip-set instead. A good tip is to stand with your back against a wall while doing this movement. This eliminates the chance for cheating. What I do instead of cheating is use a strip-set. This is sort of a self-spotting method and fully fatigues the muscle better than any cheating could. When you can't do anymore just drop the weight around 20 lbs and continue with perfect form; remember that you can do this with any movement!

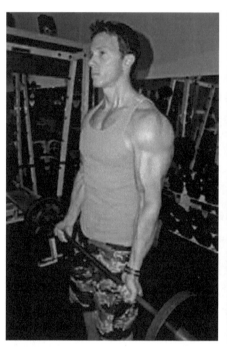 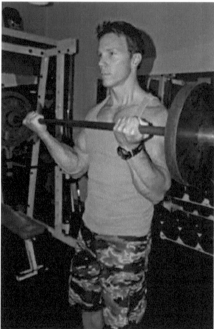

Figure 15: Barbell Curl - Starting Position    Figure 16: Barbell Curl - Ending Position

## ALTERNATE BICEPS CURL

Hold a weight in each hand, arms hanging naturally, with your elbows at your side, palms facing the sides of your thighs. The back is straight and shoulders pulled back. Begin to curl your right arm up first, exhaling while keeping the elbow totally stationary. Midway through the rep, twist the wrist palm up (supinate). The forearm should come up just short of perpendicular to the floor. As you lower the weight back down, twist the wrist back to palms facing the thighs. Inhale a breath. Wait until the right arm goes completely down to the fully extended position then begin to curl the left arm.

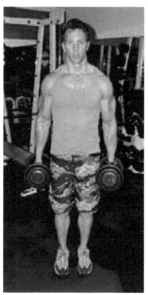 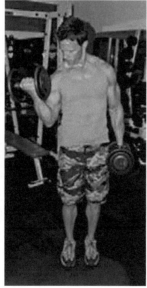 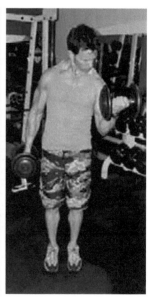

Figure 17: Barbell Curl - 1    Figure 18: Barbell Curl  - 2    Figure 19: Barbell Curl – 3

## BODYWEIGHT CURLS (INCLINE)

I'm using the Smith Machine for this movement but you can use a squat rack bar or any other solid foundation that will support your bodyweight. Using the heels as the pivot point and keeping your body rigidly straight, grasp the bar with the arms about 90 degrees to your body. Using the biceps, curl yourself up toward the bar, with the forehead coming close to touching at the top of the rep. It's important to not move the elbows down during this movement and use the back to pull yourself up. We save that movement for bodyweight rows! Slowly lower yourself back to down. To increase bodyweight, lower the bar. To decrease bodyweight, raise it.

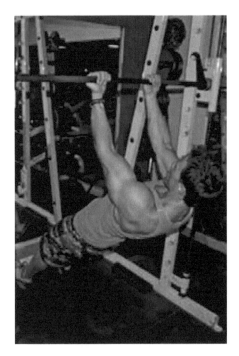

Figure 20: Incline Bodyweight Curl -
Starting Position

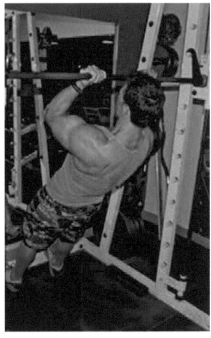

Figure 21: Incline Bodyweight Curl -
Ending Position

## INCLINE DUMBBELL CURLS

This exercise really focuses on the brachii, the primary elbow flexor when the forearm is supinated. Seat yourself in an incline bench much like you are readying for a set of incline dumbbell press; only make the incline steeper at around 50-60 degrees. From here allow the arms to hang down naturally where gravity is pulling them and keep them straight. Now, with the elbows stationary and palms facing your legs curl the weights up and twist the palms towards the ceiling as you curl them. Hold for one second and get a two-second count back down to the fully extended arm position.

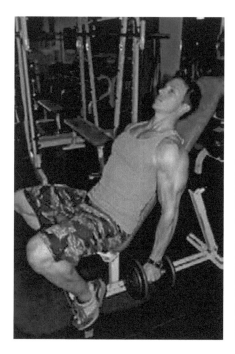 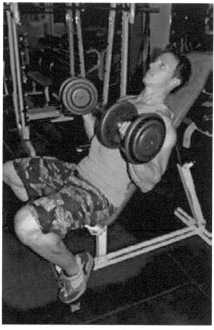

Figure 22: Incline Dumbbell Curl - Starting Position

Figure 23: Incline Dumbell Curl - Ending Position

## HAMMER CURLS

This is a great upper-arm movement. Start by holding a dumbbell in each hand towards the top of the handle as this will allow you to hold the weights much easier. With the shoulders dropped and arms hanging naturally at your sides, begin to curl the weights upward at the same time to chin height keeping the elbows secure at your sides. Keep the stress on the biceps by not coming up too high. Slowly lower them back down to the starting position and fully extend the arms at the bottom.

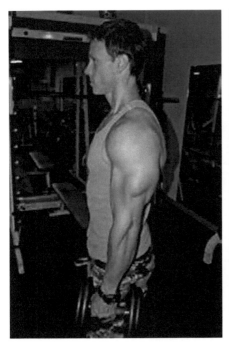 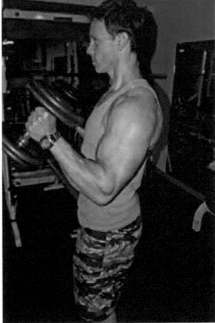

Figure 24: Hammer Curl - Starting Position    Figure 25: Hammer Curl - Ending Position

## SEATED ROW CABLE CURLS

This exercise is a change of pace from regular preacher curls and makes a great substitute in your arm routine. Attach an easy curl bar to the cable attachment. Sit upright with the on the bench with the knees bent about 90 degrees and the heels up high on the footplates. Position the elbows on the insides of each knee.

From here, grasp the curl the bar and curl it toward your head keeping back straight and the elbows as stationary as possible; elbows constantly in contact with your knees. As with any movement it's important to fully extend the arms for the best possible ROM.

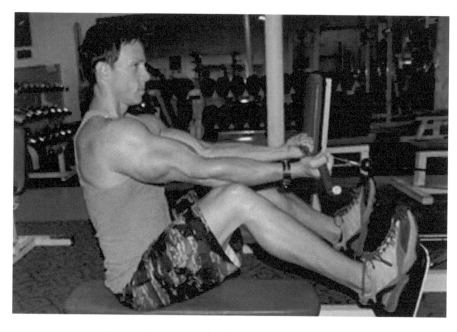

Figure 26: Seated Cable Cable Curl - Starting Position

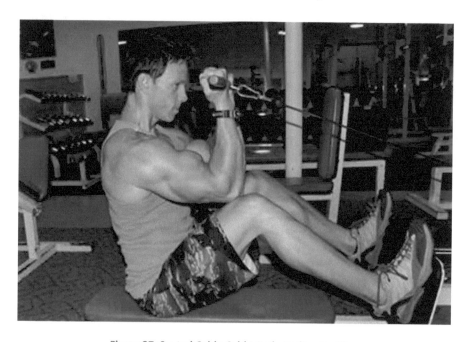

Figure 27: Seated Cable Cable Curl - Ending Position

## UPPER BODY - TRICEPS (all movements are IM's)

### TRICEPS KICKBACKS

You can either perform this exercise standing, using both arms at a time, or for added stability and focus you can do one arm at a time. I prefer to do both arms at a time while standing in the bent-over-row position. It's a more active way to do this movement and makes the heart pump harder.

Keeping the back as straight as possible, secure the elbows to the sides of the body at 90 degrees. Using only the triceps, move the weights behind you while not moving the shoulder joint. At the top of the movement (B) the arms should be close to the angle of the back. Bring the weight back down to the starting position for another rep. Make sure you don't move the elbow from your side on the way back down; the beginning elbow position is 45 degrees, never less.

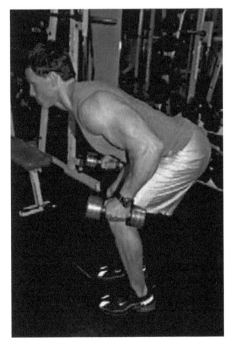 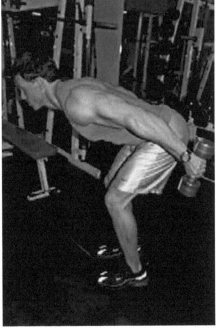

Figure 28: Triceps Kickback - Starting Position

Figure 29: Triceps Kickback - Ending Position

## OVERHEAD TRICEPS EXTENSION

This exercise hits the biggest part of the arm, the triceps, which covers 2/3 of the mass of the upper arm. Overlap and cross the hands over the dumbbell wrapping the thumbs around the grip. We are targeting the triceps with this movement so to achieve this keep your elbows as close to the sides of your head as possible. This ensures a proper stretch and helps you to not recruit your shoulders into the movement, which is important for the muscles to get stronger and more visible.

Start by raising the weight above your head almost fully extending your arms. Then slowly lower the weight to the base of the neck. You must keep your arms perpendicular to the floor throughout the entire movement. This also ensures the best stretch possible.

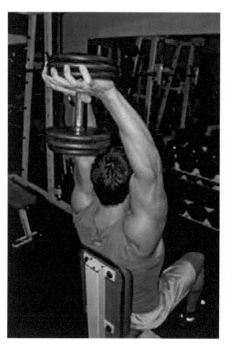 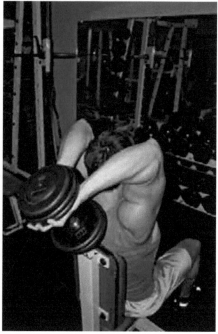

Figure 30: Triceps Extension - Starting Position

Figure 31: Triceps Extension - Ending Position

**LYING TRICEPS EXTENSION (aka head knockers, head crushers, skull crushers)**

Don't let the slang terms scare you- this is a great arm builder! Grab the bar with the hands approximately 3 to 4 inches apart and lye back on a flat bench. Lying down, press the bar up with the arms straight then tilt them back about 2 inches. With the elbows close together, lower the weight slowly to the top to the head, inhaling a breath then raise back up to the starting position while exhaling, not moving the shoulders at all. Pretend the elbows are tied together to not move them at all.

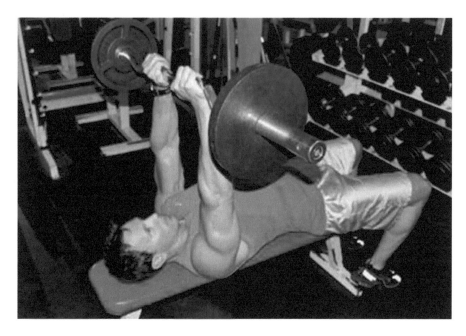

Figure 32: Lying Triceps Extension - Starting Position

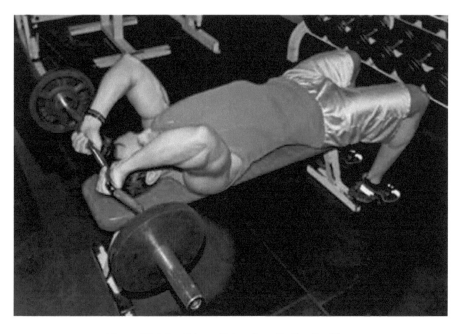

Figure 33: Lying Triceps Extension - Ending Position

## CABLE TRICEPS PUSHDOWNS

This isolation exercise works the triceps on the outside portion of the arm- the lateral head and is great bringing out that "horseshoe" look as some call it. Stand facing the machine with your hands on the bar and your elbows at your sides. Inhale and straighten your arms, but don't separate your elbows from your sides. Exhale as you press the bar down. If you use a heavier weight, put one foot out in front of your body and lean forward a bit to give yourself more stability.

There are a few variations you can perform to change it up such as supinated grip (palms up) or ropes, which allow you to get more of a peak contraction by separating the hands at the end of the movement. Which is the same as regular pushdowns, only with the palms up. This hand position doesn't allow you to use heavy weight. Just focus on your form and the medial head of the triceps will be hit effectively. (In this photo I'm using a supinated, or palms-up grip)

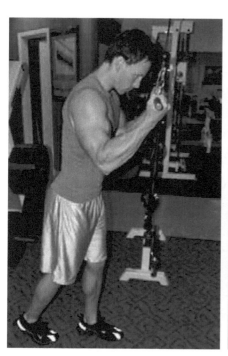

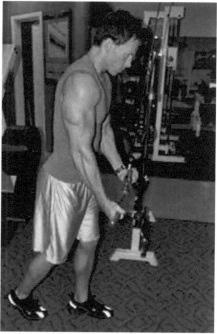

Figure 34: Triceps Pushdown - Starting Position

Figure 35: Triceps Pushdown - Ending Position

## ONE ARM CABLE PUSHDOWN

I like this one particularly as a finishing exercise because you can focus on each tricep individually. Stand facing the machine and grab the handle with an underhand grip. Keeping the elbow tight and your side, push the weight down to your thigh, exhaling. Inhale as you bring it back up.

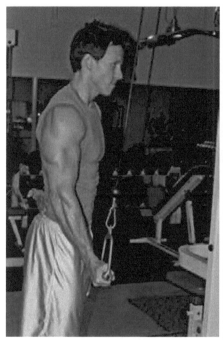 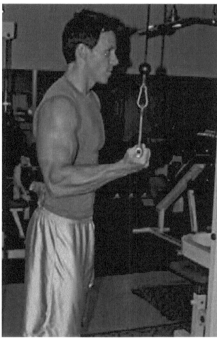

Figure 36: One Arm Cable Pushdown - Ending Position

Figure 37: One Arm Cable Pushdown - Starting Position

## DUMBBELL TRICEPS EXTENSION

Lie flat on a bench holding a dumbbell in each hand with your arms extended straight up from the shoulders. Inhale as you lower the weights down towards the sides of your head. Push them back up to the starting exhaling a breath. It's important to not move the shoulders at all and keep the arms parallel throughout the entire movement. The only thing we want moving here are the forearms. This exercise equally works all three heads of the triceps very effectively. For added intensity, tip the arms back a couple of inches. This puts more stress on the triceps.

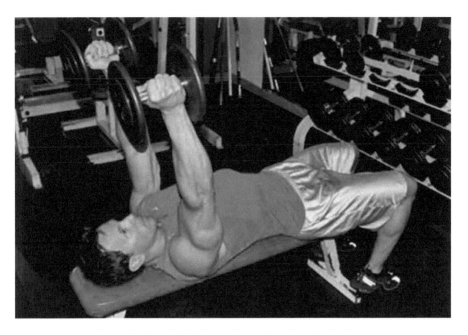

Figure 38: Dumbbell Triceps Extension - Starting Position

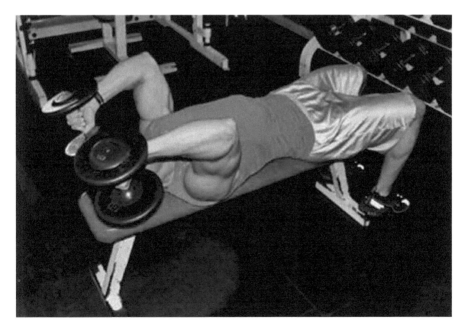

Figure 39: Dumbbell Triceps Extension - Ending Position

## UPPER BODY - BACK (all movements are IM's)

### LAT PULL DOWN

This is a welcome alternative to pull-ups and targets the lats, or the outside muscles of the upper back. Start with the knee pads set high enough allowing you to comfortably have your heels placed on the ground, but low and snug enough to not allow the weight to lift you from the seat. You may grip thumb under or over, which ever is more comfortable. Lean back slightly. Keep the back erect and the torso stationary while pulling the bar down smoothly touching the top of the chest.

The elbows should be pulled behind the line of the back. Exhale during this phase of the movement. Slowly raise the bar back up to the top allowing a nice stretch, with the shoulder blades rolling out comfortably. Inhale during this phase. Don't turn this movement into a triceps pushdown. Pull it to the upper chest and back up for reps.

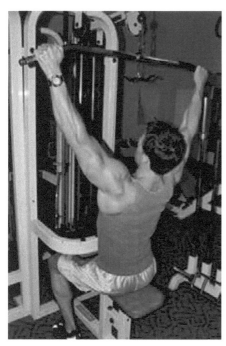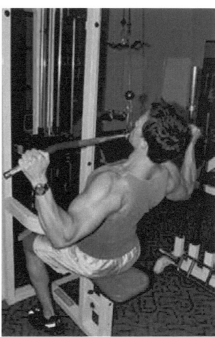

Figure 40: Lat Pull Down - Starting Position    Figure 41: Lat Pull Down - Ending Position

## BENT-OVER ROW

This exercise is very effective in targeting the middle of the back Start by placing your feet a foot or so apart, feet and knees both facing forward. Grip the bar palms up with the hands just outside the knees. Keep the back erect and the knees slightly bent. Let the arms hang naturally while holding the bar. From this starting position pull the bar to the lower abdomen keeping the elbows close to the body. Exhale as you pull. Return to the starting position, inhaling a breath.

As a variation, use dumbbells. With one in each hand, each side of the back is worked independently, forcing you to focus more intensely on proper form. It is very important to never round-out the back while doing any variation of the bent over row. You can perform these seated or standing; standing is obviously more difficult but a better place to start for getting the form correct.

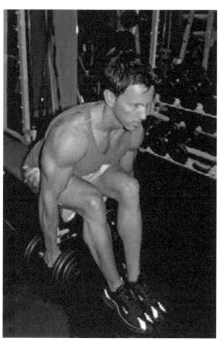 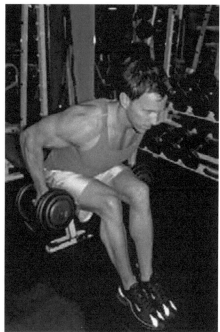

Figure 42: Bent Over Row - Starting Position     Figure 43: Bent Over Row - Ending Position

## SEATED CABLE ROW

Sit with your back totally straight and not hunched over in the least. It's extremely important to have your back engaged and straight during this movement. Place your feet firmly on the footplates with the knees bent slightly. Row the weight back almost to touch your waistline. Keep the elbows in close to the body, touch the grip to your shirt and slowly lower it back to the starting position. Remember to inhale during the pull phase and exhale during the return phase of the movement.

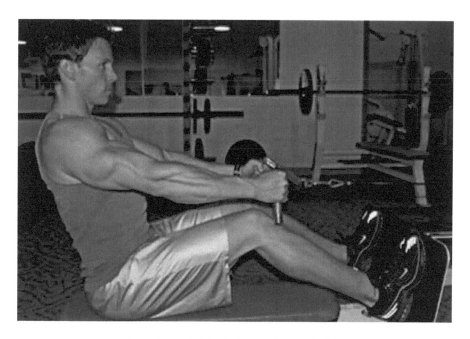

Figure 44: Seated Cable Row – Starting Position

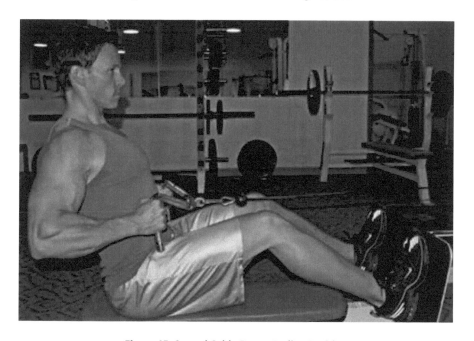

Figure 45: Seated Cable Row – Ending Position

## UPPER BODY - SHOULDERS

### UPRIGHT ROWS

Begin by placing the feet no wider than shoulder width apart with the knees bent slightly. Straighten the arms and grip the bar with a few inches between the hands. Without touching the body, raise the bar slowly to the chin with the elbows raised up high around the ears. The hands should not be higher than the elbows. Again, without touching the body, lower the bar slowly to return the arms to the fully extended starting position and repeat the repetition.

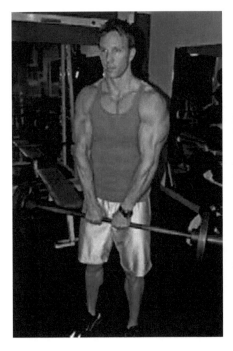 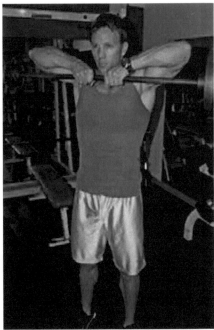

Figure 46: Upright Row – Starting Position     Figure 47: Upright Row – Ending Position

## LATERAL RAISES

Place the feet a few inches apart, with the knees bent slightly. Keep the back erect as you lean forward slightly. With the weights in front of your thighs, begin to slowly raise them up. As you raise them slightly bend the elbows and tilt the weights inward as if you were pouring a pitcher of water. Bring your arms up just past parallel level to the floor. Slowly lower the weights back to the starting position in front of the thighs. Repeat.

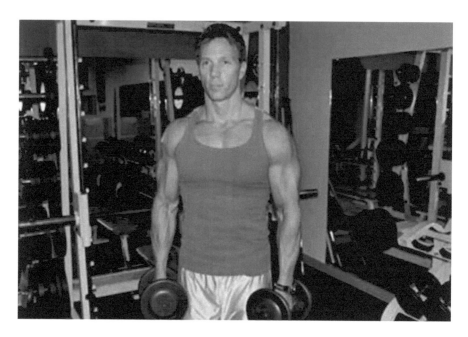

Figure 48: Lateral Raises - Starting Position

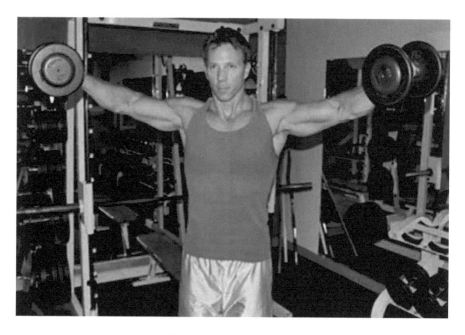

Figure 49: Lateral Raises - Ending Position

## MILITARY PRESSES

This is the most basic and common of the shoulder exercises. Start with the hands placed far enough apart to where the forearms are parallel to each other. Slowly lower the weight to the FRONT of the body, very close to the face, touching the bar to the upper chest. Raise the bar back to the upright position with the arms extended. Repeat. It is recommended that you use some sort of back support or bench while performing this exercise to give extra support but it's not necessary. If you don't have that support, try to use a lighter weight.

(Military Presses with Dumbbells)   Start with the weights on your knees. Pulling with the biceps, kick them up to the starting position one at a time. Forearms parallel to each other, begin to press them overhead, not touching the weights at the top. Arms are fully extended. Hold for a second count then lower the bar back down for a two-second count back to starting position.

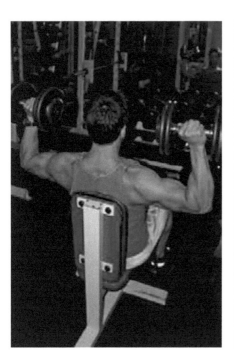

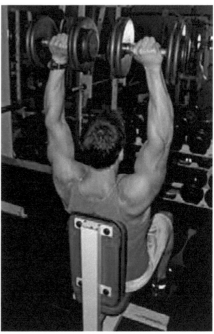

Figure 50: Military Presses - Starting
Position

Figure 51: Military Presses - Ending
Position

## LOWER BODY - LEGS

Leg training is a staple of fat-burning capacity for our bodies and this means seeing Abs! The muscles of the legs are very large and have many muscle fibers that are metabolically active and require more calories burned to efficiently train them. The take home message? Train your legs to see your Abs!! Take this very seriously, leg training can change your body unlike any other muscle group can especially at the onset of your program. Let's cover these powerful fat-burning movements. When we combine the compound leg movements into supersets with other movements, look out. Your results will almost be fail-safe.

### BARBELL SQUAT (CM)

By most experts' standards, the squat is the king of all exercises for total leg development. Start by placing your feet shoulder width, placing the bar across your upper back, (middle of the shoulder blades) and hold it there steadily with the arms at a comfortable placement on the bar. It is extremely important that you keep your back erect or arched from beginning to the end of this movement. Slowly begin the squat, placing pressure on the heels not letting the knees pass over the toes. Your thighs should not go past parallel to the floor. The entire rep range should be slow and controlled. Inhale as you descend and exhale as you go back up.

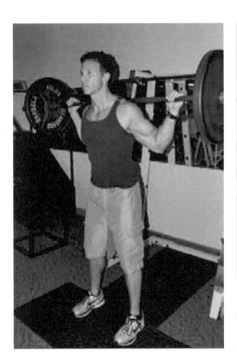
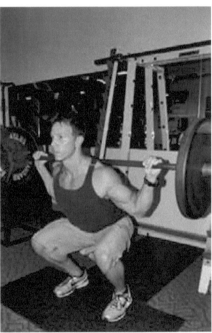

Figure 52: Barbell Squat - Starting Position   Figure 53: Barbell Squat – Ending Position

## DUMBELL LUNGE (CM)

This exercise focuses on the largest muscles in the body, your glutes (your butt) and also hits the quads in the front of the legs as well. Hold a dumbbell in each hand, arms hanging at your sides. Step out with one leg while keeping the back straight. You must step out far enough so that the knee does not pass over the toe. This puts too much stress on the knee. Go down far enough so that on the trailing leg the opposite knee nearly touches the ground. Keep this stance and repeat this for your repetitions. I have found it is safer and easier on the knees to do each leg as a complete set and not alternate steps. Why? I have seen people stepping forward for the "walking lunge" and strain their knee. The reason for this is simple: Not only are you resisting the weight of your own body on one knee and possibly added weight of the dumbbells but you are also multiplying that many times over with the momentum of the step. It is far safer and just as effective to not employ a stepping lunge and just do each leg for reps at a time.

Variations include a regular bar on your back, the smith machine (my personal favorite with one leg propped up on a bench) it makes the movement that much tougher and more effective because your trailing leg can't be used as easily to cheat by helping the working leg- this variation works the glutes more effectively than any other movement I have used. I will say again that this movement is one of the most challenging my clients or myself for that matter have done when it comes to difficulty and effectiveness. Each time I do these I feel like I have just run a 200 meter sprint.

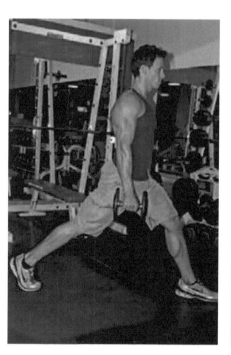

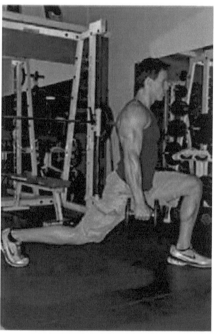

Figure 54: Dumbbell Lunge - Starting
Position

Figure 55: Dumbbell Lunge – Ending
Position

## STIFF-LEGGED DEAD LIFT (HAMSTRINGS)

This exercise involves all of the spinal erectors and stretches the hamstrings very effectively. In fact, no other exercise produces healthy hamstring soreness better than these. You can use a barbell or hold dumbbells in each hand. Start by holding the weight close to your thighs, almost touching them. Slowly begin to bend over, keeping the knees locked and bent slightly. Keep the weight close to the body- this protects the back. The back MUST stay erect. A good way to keep the back straight is to actually stick your rear end out, sounds goofy but it works.

Go down as far as you comfortably can, as you will begin to feel the pull in your hamstrings as you lower the weights to the ground. Slowly return to the starting position. Due to the stress put on the lumbar, it is probably a good idea to use relatively light weight while doing this movement if you are new to it. As always however try to challenge yourself by adding weight as you progress. This increases intensity and Ultimate results!

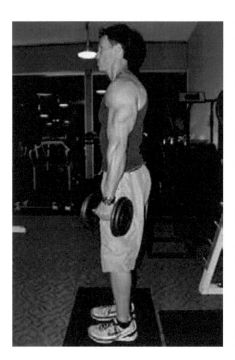
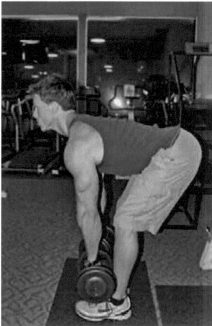

Figure 56: Stiff-Legged Deadlift - Starting Position

Figure 57: Stiff-Legged Deadlift – Ending Position

## ANGLED LEG PRESS

This machine is a great alternative to squats if you have any sort of back problem.  Adjust the back pad to fit your height- the taller you are, the more reclined it should be and vice versa.  Sit in the machine, lying back against the angled back pad. Some of the pads have lower back support, others don't. If they don't, just use a towel folded to the desired thickness. Place the feet midway on the platform, about shoulder width apart. To target the front thighs the feet should be placed lower on the platform. Conversely, to target the hamstrings/glutes more intensely, place your feet higher.

Inhale, raise the carriage up off of the pegs and lock them out. Slowly lower the weight, keeping the pressure on the heels of the feet.  Lower the carriage toward your chest while letting the knees travel to the sides of the chest. It is very important to keep your but on the pad at all times.

When your thighs touch the bottom of your ribcage, you have gone down far enough. Slowly push the carriage back up, make sure you DON'T lock your knees at the top.

*Variation- Perform these one leg at a time. This offers a different option in place of lunges to keep mixing it up! Do them as if you had both feet on the plate; keeping each leg on its separate side. Some days you just don't feel like doing leg movements with weight on your back. This is a great way to do just that, effectively.

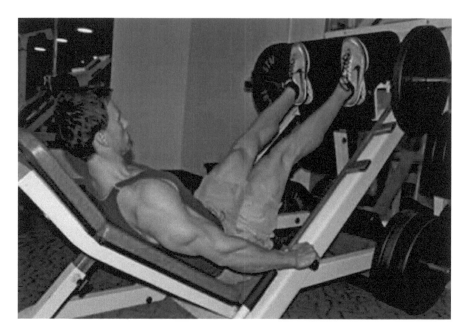

Figure 58: Angled Leg Press - Starting Position

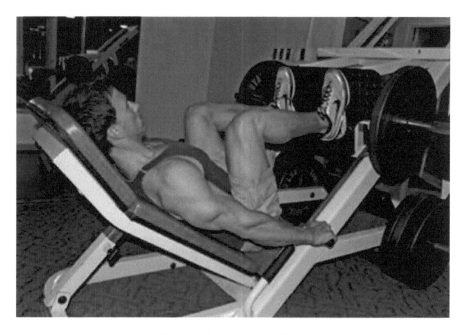

Figure 59: Angled Leg Press - Ending Position

84

## SIDE LUNGE

Begin with feet spread apart (a comfortable stretching distance) and cross the arms high on the across the chest. Angle the feet outward slightly. Depending on how your knees feel or the shape they are in, angle the feet to suit your comfort level. Everyone's knees feel different on various movements so it's important to customize.

From this position, squat down on one leg, keeping your weight on the heel. Go down as far as it's comfortable. To make this exercise more effective, lower yourself as far as you can go. A longer lunge puts focus more on the glutes, a shorter lunge puts focus on the quads. When you are ready, use extra weight by holding dumbbells at your sides. I routinely use this movement super-setted with heavier leg presses or squats.

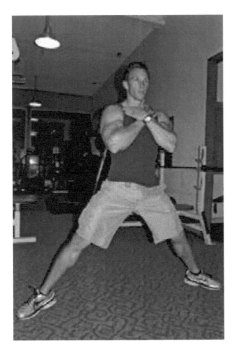
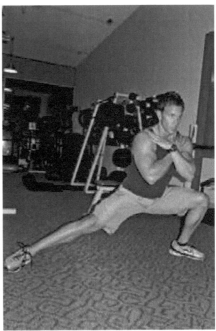

Figure 60: Side Lunge - Starting Position    Figure 61: Side Lunge - Ending Position

## STABILITY BALL HAMSTRING CURLS

Start by placing your calves on the top of the stability ball, lying with your back on the ground. Begin the movement by making the body as rigid and straight-line as possible. Curl your feet towards your butt, ending the movement with your heels on the ball. To lessen the weight, bring your butt back down closer to the floor making the body less rigid. This movement is just as effective as any bulky leg curl machine can be and more challenging!

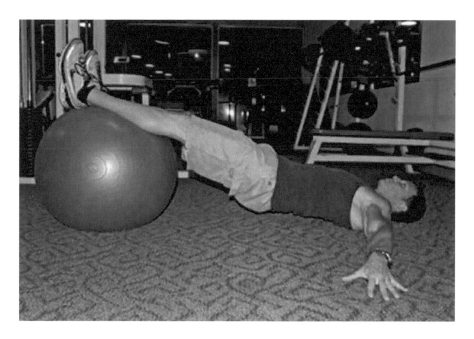

Figure 62: Stability Ball Hamstring Curl - Starting Position

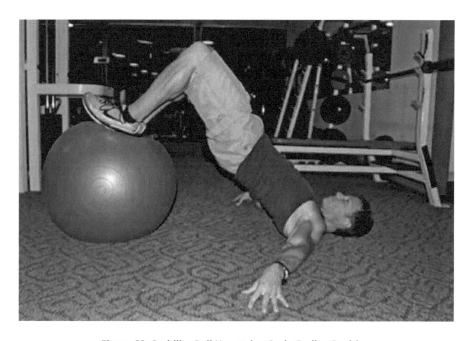

Figure 63: Stability Ball Hamstring Curl - Ending Position

# LOWER BODY - CALVES (lower leg)

## STANDING CALF RAISE

Some gyms have this machine, others do not. If they don't, no worries. I just do them one leg at a time. The weight of the body on each calf individually will provide enough weight and intensity. The important points to remember are don't move your knees while doing this movement and don't lock your knees but keep them slightly bent just above lockout. The only joint moving during the motion is the ankle. Get up high enough on a solid surface or block and proceed to lower the heels down to the ground, getting a great stretch in the calf muscle.

This movement focuses on the gastrocnemius muscle, the one toward the inside of the leg giving it that "diamond" shape. Whenever standing, this muscle is the primary mover to extend the foot. Press back up to the top, keeping the pressure on the balls of the feet. Some experts say you should angle the feet in or out to target different areas of the calves but I disagree with that theory as it can place undue stress on the knees. If you want to do this, just put the pressure on the outside of the feet near the little to- while keeping the feet inline and parallel to each other. It's important to keep your weight straight up and down above your heals so don't lean forward! The exercise won't be as effective.

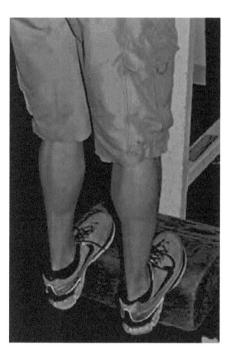

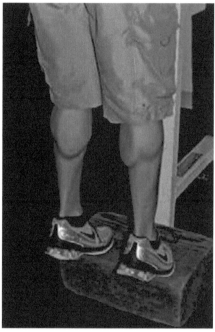

Figure 64: Standing Calf Raise - Starting Position

Figure 65: Standing Calf Raise - Ending Position

## SEATED CALF RAISE

This movement focuses on the soleus muscle of the calf, or what looks to be the outer portion of the lower leg. When the knee is bent at 90% or we are seated, this muscle is the primary mover and extends the foot. Get into position on the seat, put the knees under the pads not cheating by using leverage of too much leg. Keep the pads just passed the kneecaps to keep this movement honest and effective. The same rules apply to this movement as standing calf raises- keep the balls of the feet as the main pressure points and slowly lower the heels to the floor. Come up slowly and repeat for reps. The gastrocnemius does help as a secondary mover.

*Tip: For each of the previous movements, there are different ways to do them- as in confuse your muscles for results. Different tools create new stimuli and your muscles get confused. The cable station is a prime example. Clip different tools to the cable station and you have a different exercise, for the most part. It's a different feel and the muscle responds in an effective way to cope with the "new" stress. Example- standing barbell curls can be done at the cable station with various grips. You don't always have to do the same exercises. Do them differently with new tools, angles and set schemes. You'll see how in Chapter 5.

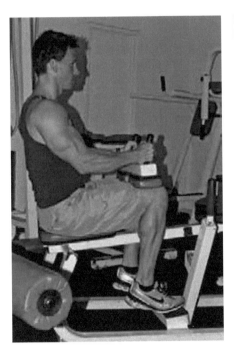

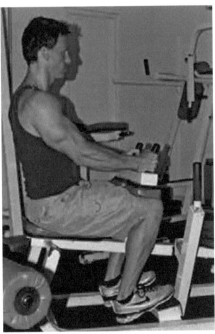

Figure 66: Seated Calf Raise - Starting Position

Figure 67: Seated Calf Raise - Ending Position

## AWESOME ABS- MY FAVORITE AB CARVING MOVEMENTS

Remember all that talk about how you don't need to do all those endless sets of crunches and/or sit-ups to get your Abs to come out? Well it's true you don't. What you do need to do is supplement your regular training with the following movements for ultimate Abs, to put a refining touch on the look you really want. Further, doing some AB work will help strengthen and protect your back. As I mentioned before, Abs are like any other muscle group. If trained with direct intensity they must be rested. These movements you're about to learn are very effective in that they are high intensity and don't allow you to do "endless sets". Some of these movements require the use of an exercise ball- (aka Swiss or physio-ball) the big inflatable balls you sometimes see in the gyms. They are effective, hard hitting and will yield you great results so they are worth doing. They will actually help you chisel out the flat, hard squares if that's the look you want. If not, you can always scale back the intensity and not implement these exercises.


## AB FAVORITES

### HANGING LEG RAISES (I call them 45's)

These are #1 as they are the most challenging for me to do and thus really get me amazing results. Start as a regular hanging leg raise, get in the straps and begin to curl your knees up to your chest. Go up as high as you can, also by curling your lower back and butt into the movement at the top. The twist is- don't go back down all the way. You're going to stop with your thighs parallel to the floor-that's your rep. Now curl the knees back up to the chest and continue at a quick but controlled pace. For a real burn, do as many of these as you can then rep out with regular lower half leg raises. Your Abs will be on fire and before you know it, you will start to see lower Abs develop and that elusive awesome "V" taper at the waistline that men and women both like.

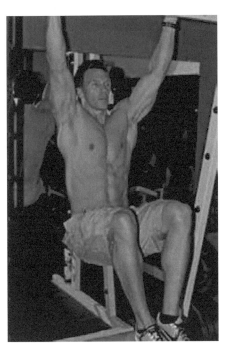 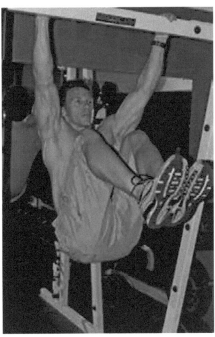

Figure 68: Hanging Leg Raises - Starting Position

Figure 69: Hanging Leg Raises - Ending Position

## SIDE BRIDGES

One of the best abdominal and back strengtheners. There are different variations for difficulty of this movement. Let's start with the easiest.

- **Bent-knee side bridge-** Lie on your side with your forearm on the floor and your elbow under your shoulder, your knees bent at 90 degrees. Keep your glutes and Abs tight throughout the ROM. Raise your hips off the ground until your torso is straight from shoulders to knees. Repeat it for reps. For a kicker at the end, hold the rep up off the ground for as long as you can.

- **Full side bridge-** You can probably deduct this one is the full version of the fore mentioned. Use your feet staggered as the pivot point. You're supporting more of your weight this way so prepare to feel it!

- **Elevated side bridge-** Use this one when full side bridges get too easy! Same as the full side bridge, but place your feet higher than your shoulders. Doesn't matter how high really, that depends on how much resistance you want. Use a block, a chair, anything to elevate your legs and don't allow your hips to droop.

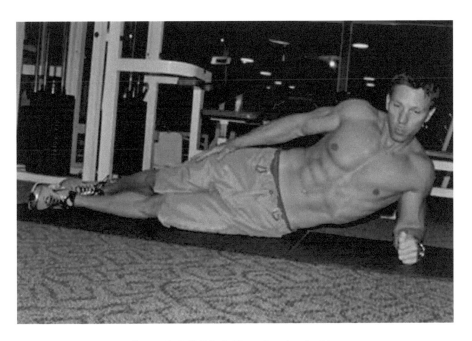

Figure 70: Full Side Bridge - Starting Position

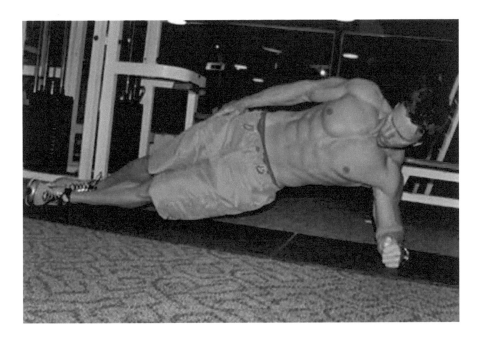

Figure 71: Full Side Bridge - Ending Position

## STABILITY BALL CRUNCHES (MODIFIED)

These are so basic yet so effective. Most of the basics are! I do them super-setted with the hanging leg raises for an all-out assault on my Abs when I feel like it. I do them first with my hands across my chest as an easier, lighter set. The second set I will extend my arms straight and out over my head. Your arms actually weight quite a bit providing great resistance while doing these.

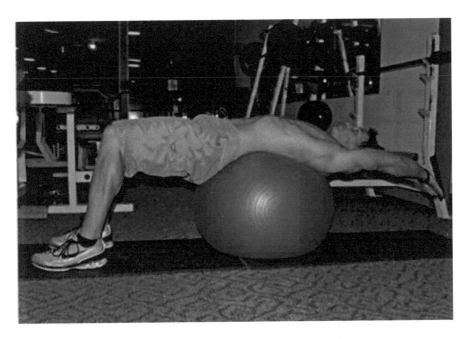

Figure 72: Stability Ball Crunch - Starting Position

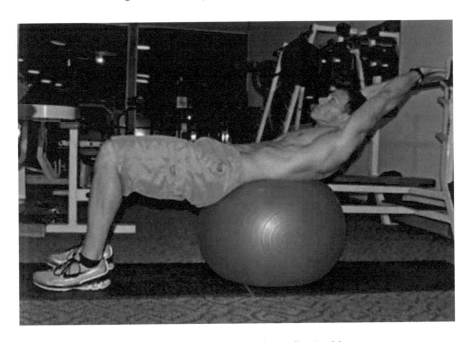

Figure 73: Stability Ball Crunch - Ending Position

## STABILITY BALL HANDOFF

Lie flat on your back, handing the ball off to your feet as you bring your hands and legs together at the top. Bring your shoulders off the floor as you make the handoff until you can't anymore. Repeat the handoff again to your hands and bring the ball back down to the starting position. Don't touch the floor!

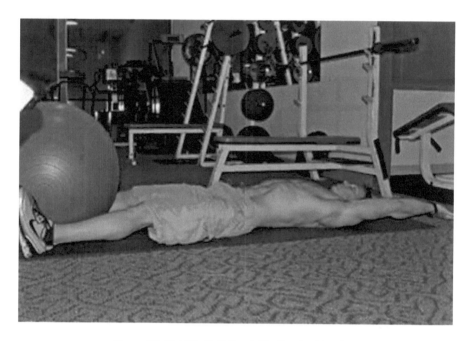

Figure 74: Stability Ball Handoff - Starting Position

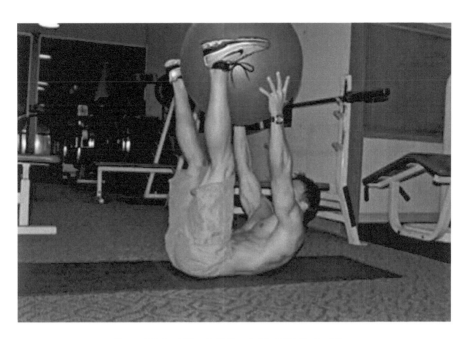

Figure 75: Stability Ball Handoff – Middle Position

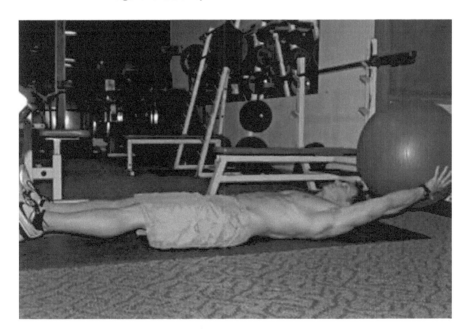

Figure 76: Stability Ball Handoff - Ending Position

## CIRCLE LEG LIFTS

Lie flat on your back, legs up, feet together straight at 90 degrees to the hip. Make a circle with your legs, holding your legs up. Hold a couple dumbbells for stability.

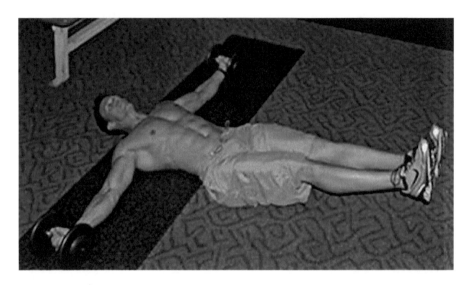

Figure 77: Circle Leg Lifts - Starting Position

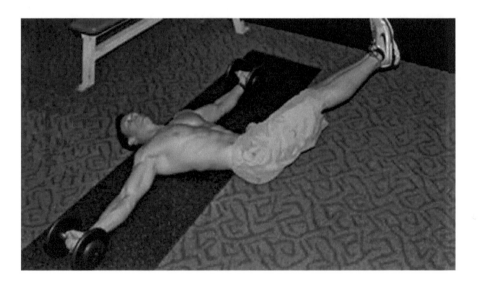

Figure 78: Circle Leg Lifts – Second Position

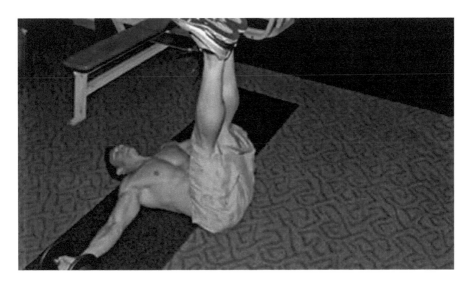

Figure 79: Circle Leg Lifts - Third Position

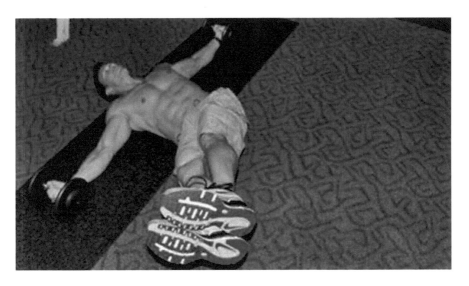

Figure 80: Circle Leg Lifts - Ending Position

## HANGING HALF MOONS

Like my favorite hanging leg raises, start these from the same position in straps or hanging on with your hands. Instead of frontal lifts, bring your knees full circle and back again for one full rep. This one is very challenging and works the entire abdominal wall as well as the oblique regions. It is also a great lumbar rotation movement.

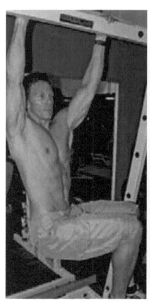 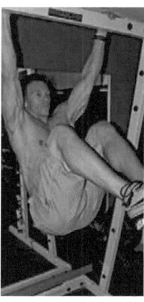 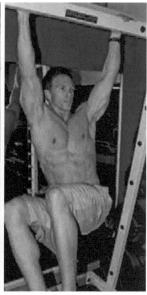

Figure 81: Hanging Half Moons Starting Position

Figure 82: Hanging Half Moons Second Position

Figure 83: Hanging Half Moons Ending Position

## STABILITY BALL REVERSE CRUNCHES

Lie flat on your back on the floor. Put the ball between your knees and heels of your feet holding it there snugly. Place your arms beside you on the floor palms down. Using your Abs, pick the ball up off the floor and lift your butt and lower back up off the floor. Go back down slowly the starting position. This completes a rep.

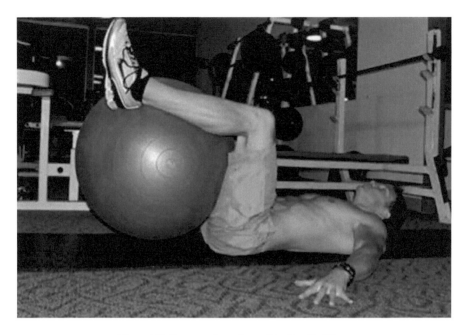

Figure 84: Reverse Crunches – Starting Position

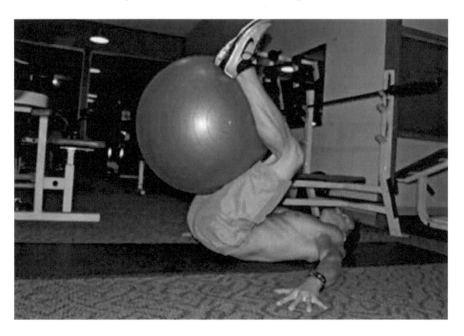

Figure 85: Reverse Crunches – Ending Position

## ROLLOUTS

Lay down a towel for padding and go down on both knees. Use a wheel designed for this movement or an Olympic-style bar with round weights on each side. Five or ten pound weights will do. Lean forward slightly, keeping the back straight and grasp the bar. Slowly roll forward as far as you can comfortably go pushing the bar as far out forward as you can with your arms straight. Warning: prepare to be challenged!

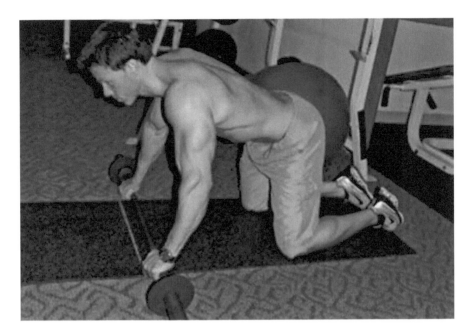

Figure 86: Rollouts - Starting Position

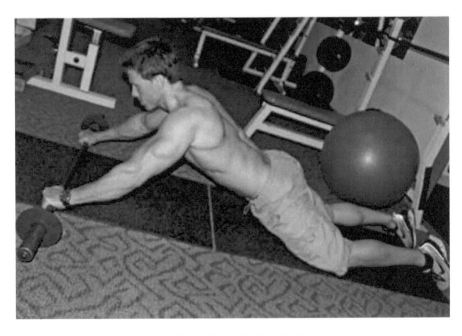

Figure 87: Rollouts - Ending Position

## STABILITY BALL PRONE KNEE TUCKS

Start by relaxing on the ball on your stomach- enjoy it while it lasts. From here, roll forward and catch yourself with your hands on the ground in pushup position. While keeping your body as rigid as possible, inch ahead until the ball is in contact with your shins just under the knees. Tighten the Abs, bring the knees up to the chest. This one is tougher because it calls you to balance and hold yourself up in the push-up position throughout the whole movement and the Abs are constantly contracting to keep your body rigid. You will feel it in your shoulders, triceps and chest as these all assist in keeping you steady. When you get this down try a more advanced one leg at-a-time. Just keep one shin in contact with the ball and let the other semi-tucked out of the way of the ball. Try for as many as you can on each leg.

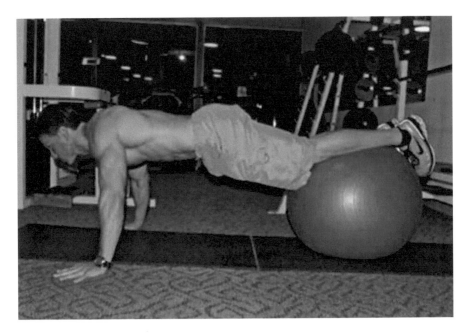

Figure 88: Prone Knee Tucks – Starting Position

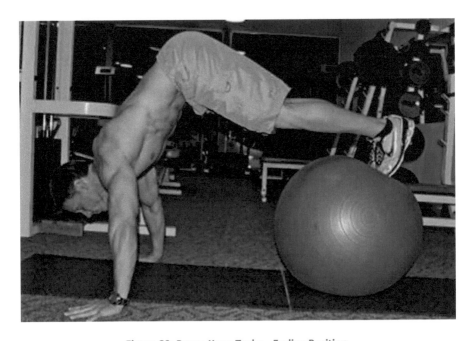

Figure 89: Prone Knee Tucks – Ending Position

## Combined Movements for Ultimate Fat Burning

These movements are designed to have muscle groups work together in one combined movement for increased heart rate, fat burning and results. For these reasons they work best for those who need to lose extra body fat and inches. You generally must use a lighter weight with these movements as your energy is being tapped on many different muscles in one fluid movement so you don't need heavy weight. They are equivalent to a sprint in terms of your energy output in a short, focused amount of time.

### SQUAT TO SHOULDER PRESS

A staple combo-compound movement. Starting in the standing position with dumbbells in the starting position at the sides of your head, lower into a full squat position and rise back up to the top. Once back up, push the weights to the ceiling, lower them back down while simultaneously going back down into another full squat.

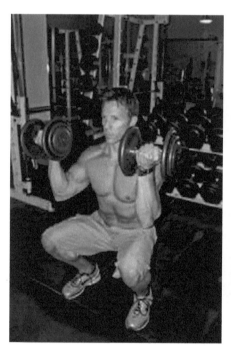

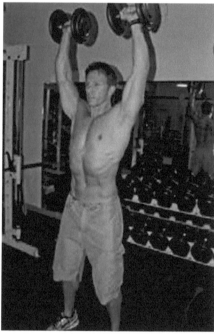

Figure 90: Squat to Shoulder Press - Starting Position

Figure 91: Squat to Shoulder Press - Ending Position

## SQUAT TO BICEP CURL TO SHOULDER PRESS

Three movements: Two compound and one isolation. You can use a barbell or a dumbbell for this movement, the only difference being dumbbells are more versatile and can be held at your sides vs. a bar which would have you begin from a dead-lift position.

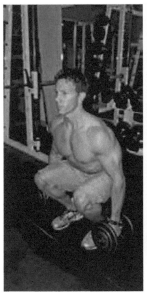 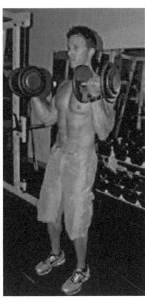 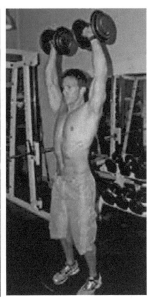

Figure 92: Squat          Figure 93: Bicep Curl          Figure 94: Shoulder Press

## LUNGES TO UPRIGHT ROWS

Using the ultra-effective lunge, dumbbells at your sides, as you come up to the top of your motion begin the upright rows. Lower the weights as you go back down. Hit each leg separately- this allows more intensity.

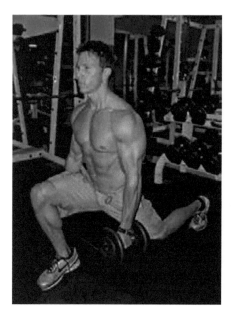 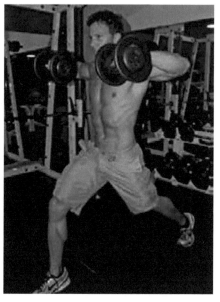

Figure 95: Lunge to Upright Row – Starting Position

Figure 96: Lunge to Upright Row – Ending Position

## *Stretch for results!*

It used to be commonplace to perform some stretching before exercise. How you train and with what is however a big factor in when you should stretch. Now it is more understood that stretching during (between sets) and after your weight training workouts do more to help avoid injury and post-workout soreness. The thinking here is that if you stretch before you train your muscles or joints/connective tissues could possibly get too loose and more prone to being pulled or injured. The following are stretching movements I perform during my lifting sessions targeted to each muscle group I am working at that time. Key points: Relax the muscle! No bouncing, slow and controlled, hold the stretches for 30-45 seconds, never pull too hard and only go for slight tension- not pain. If you have pain, stop, evaluate what kind and see your Doctor.

## CHEST

Stand with your arm parallel to the floor anchored to a solid structure like a wall or heavy machine (something that won't move) keeping the elbow straight. Take a small step forward so the anchored hand is behind you. Now, slowly turn away from the anchored hand. Hold for 30-45 seconds.

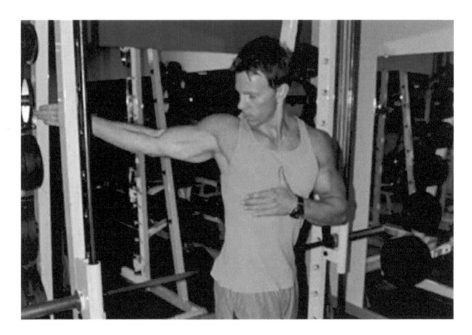

Figure 97: Chest Stretch

## BICEPS

Biceps can be done in the same fashion- Simply make a "knife edge" with your hand by tucking in the thumb and putting that edge of the hand on the anchored surface. Turn and hold in the same fashion. Some of the stretch will be placed on the bicep but you will still feel it in your chest, this is normal.

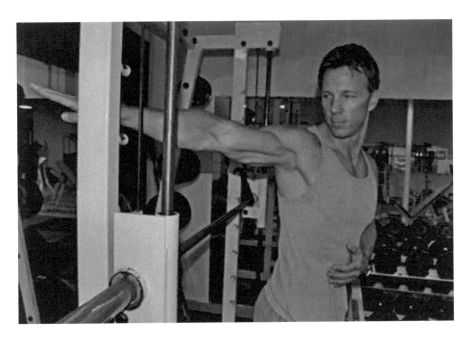

Figure 99: Biceps Stretch

## SHOULDERS

Stand with your back facing a bar or solid structure about shoulder height. Reach behind, grasping with palms up. Lean forward and bend your knees to lower and stretch your shoulders.

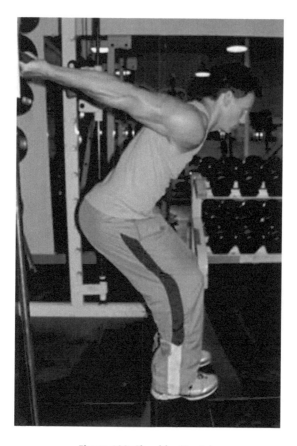

Figure 100: Shoulder Stretch

**UPPER BACK**

Hold on to a solid structure with the hands touching. Relaxing the entire back, squat down and lean back.

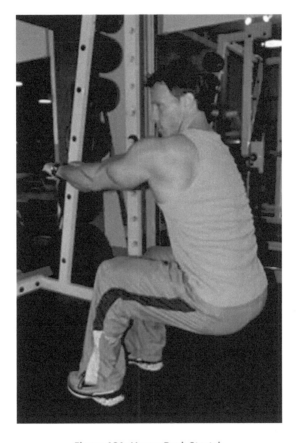

Figure 101: Upper Back Stretch

## LEGS/QUADS

Stand facing away from a bar or solid surface no more than waist high, prop on foot up on the surface (using the tongue of the shoe as the contact point) Slowly lean back to feel slight tension in the quadriceps. If you have sensitive knees use the opposite hand to opposite leg pull- just make sure you have a foundation to balance on close by.

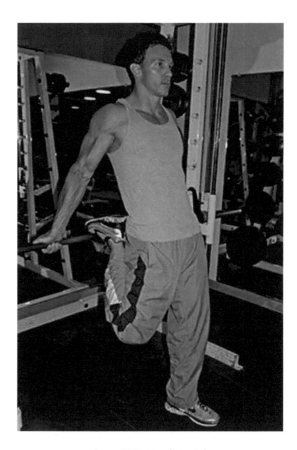

Figure 102: Quad Stretch

## LOWER BACK/LEGS

Squat down, feet shoulder width at about 15 degrees. Relaxing the hips, bring the arms inside the knees with the hands down in front of you on the floor. If you have difficulty in this position, hold on to something for support. This is a great stretch for the knees, ankles, Achilles tendons, groin, lower back and hips- which all are recruited while performing leg movements.

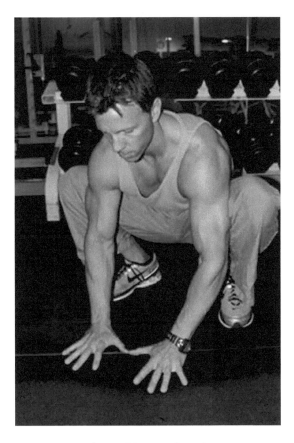

Figure 103: Squat Stretch

## LOWER BACK/HAMSTRINGS

This stretch is great for the hip flexor, hamstrings and the lower back. It's one of my favorites for relieving tension in the lower back by stretching three muscles of the iliopsoas (psoas) group. The psoas major's origin is the vertebra of the lower back and has insertion across the hip joint.

If you sit for extended periods of time (most of us do at work) the psoas group tends to get short, tight and pulls on the lower back so do this stretch! Move one leg forward until knee of your forward leg is directly over the ankle. Other knee is resting on the floor/padded surface. Now, without changing the position of knee on floor or forward foot, lower front of hip downward to create tension. Stretch both legs.

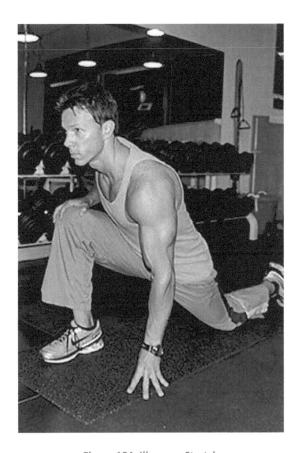

Figure 104: Iliopsoas Stretch

# CHAPTER 4: Fat Burning Cardio (My Style)

## *Sprinting vs. jogging*

In this short but informative chapter I'm going to get into some facts and opinions about cardio. I'll compare my intensive cardio method to "easier cardio"- running on a treadmill or doing a light jog outdoors. First, I want to reiterate that I'm all for doing ANY form of exercise. Doing something is better than doing nothing. I'm talking about people that I see daily who do easy cardio, but whose bodies just don't change. I see them like mice in the pin-wheel every week just treading away. If this is you, I want to invite you to try cardio and running the way I do it: short, intense and effective.

My cardio sessions are over in less than 30 minutes. I do it this way because a) I hate distance running and b) this method works better because it keeps fat-burning muscle on my frame and doesn't turn it into an energy source like distance running can do. That's why you see some of those marathoners look so skinny and unhealthy. In my eyes, jogging is virtually useless; I can only think of one good thing it can provide: a warm-up for my sprint workouts. Think of it on a natural level. Man invented jogging. He didn't do it to survive in the stone ages. No other creature in nature jogs. Animals conserve energy and walk from point A to point B or sprint as fast as they can to catch prey or avoid becoming prey themselves. You'll never see a lion or a bear jogging endlessly through their domain. They just have too much common sense for that and would rather conserve energy.

I do short, intense sprinting sessions. I think of them much like a set of bench-presses or any other movement in the gym, but the resistance is either a hill (if you can find one to run up) or the intensity you run each sprint. If I don't have a hill I will use flat ground and I'll often bring a set of weights to do supersets. You can see a complete video on how I do these here.

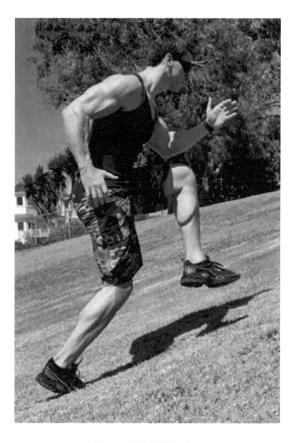

Figure 105: Hill Sprint

Find a field or a hill where you can sprint as fast as you can for a maximum of 20 seconds. Once you hit the end or reach the top, walk back and catch your breath. When you make it to the bottom, hit it again. Do this as many times as you can but if you're new to it keep the volume low- a couple will do.  If you train regularly or put your heart rate in an elevated state on a regular basis, then aim for four to six times if possible. My workout moods and energy levels vary from day to day, but I usually aim for ten to fifteen sets of sprints. If you're feeling especially strong, throw in some calisthenics as soon as you walk back down, before you start another sprint.

I have to say this will be NOTHING like jogging on a treadmill or taking a lazy jog around the block. Your lungs will be on fire, you will have a massive feeling of euphoria and a runner's high like never before. The physical results will also blow you away. You will begin to see your muscles and Abs reveal themselves from the body they have been hiding in.

Now, let's take a quick look to compare the benefits of sprinting vs. long cardio sessions as far as burning fat and getting the body of your dreams goes. You're going to love this.

One of the best features of sprinting is that it causes your body to release natural HGH – there it is again, human growth hormone. Starting to see the similarities with weight training and sprinting yet? Intensity pays huge dividends!  As we know, HGH is the fitness wonder and anti-aging hormone. Some people take synthetic shots of this stuff. If only they knew that running sprints or hill sprints increase natural HGH production by a fairly large margin. That is simply amazing. When it comes to burning fat or getting that amazing body, how can you not sprint? Even better, those high levels of HGH will remain for up to two hours after your sprint session is done. This translates to even more fat-burning for that extra amount of time, so say goodbye to stubborn belly fat!

Jogging or distance running just can't compare and does nothing even close to this. In a nutshell, sprinting builds you up, which is what getting in Ultimate shape is all about. Have a look at Olympic sprinters and then look at their distance-running counterparts. Who looks healthier? Who looks younger and more vibrant? Exactly. Sprinting builds us up and distance running tears us down. Which state would you rather be in? It's simply impossible to have an HGH producing, muscle-building, fat-incinerating, age-defying jog. Another great injury-preventing feature of hill-sprints is that when going up the hill, the elevation creates a shorter distance for your feet to travel back down to each step. Couple this with the softer surface of grass and you have another reason to feel better about sprinting hills! It's easier on your body and gets you in amazing shape in half the time.

## *What about jogging?*

Hey, don't get me wrong - it's good for your heart to jog! Just like it's good to go for a walk. Besides, your heart doesn't keep score or even know what mode of training you are putting it through. All it knows is that is beating at an increased rate for at least 20 minutes. Jogging does get your heart rate elevated. Somewhat. What it also does over time is break you down; and not in a good way. If I couldn't sprint for whatever reason I would rather speed-walk than jog. I see a lot of people out there running on the streets and sidewalks and I have to cringe. Without proper technique the pounding that real distance running is putting their bodies through is painful to watch. The knees, hips, ankles, back and neck take a beating with each step. This in itself is enough to not do it. Sadly a lot of these folks don't seem to be in that good of shape either. This is why finding a flat, solid, hole-free grass field is safer and much easier on the body for sprinting. Some cities are now installing those artificial turf fields and those are great as well. The material they use acts as a shock absorber. If you have one of those nearby, I highly recommend utilizing it. Overall, when you are running to lose inches and pounds it is probably more effective to do it first thing in the morning on a somewhat empty stomach.

Have you ever tried to run on a full stomach? Or even a stomach after drinking too much water? It's pretty gross and I can't bear the feeling I get from it. It feels like a washing machine on a spin-cycle. So, do it on an empty stomach for results. Just have something light like a half banana, and take some water with you. The potassium will help fight off muscle cramping. Sip the water when you start feeling the need, just don't overdo it.

## Treadmills vs. Running Free

What about when it's cold and rainy outside and you really want to get in your sprinting session? Looks like a treadmill day. That's okay, I think it's a good backup now and again. I try to avoid running on them, as I think they actually compromise my sprinting mechanics. The way I challenge myself for sprinting sessions makes it tough for me to get into the placid groove of a treadmill, toying with buttons to change the speed and incline. Some treadmills have automated programming and are pretty advanced but they just don't provide the raw and intense feeling of the track ahead of you or the towering hill you're about to attack.

So, back to the original thought here. When on a treadmill, lots of people change their running form and this is something you should try to avoid (unless it's needed). Unfortunately, the moving belt of the treadmill can make a mess of your running mechanics. This can be equated to working on some weight machines vs. using free weights- the body's natural arcs of range of motion are confined to the machine's tracks. The belt forces some runners to lean too far forward at the waist in an attempt to maintain or keep up with the treadmill. Others run with an extremely tight or reserved stride. Some bounce uncontrollably with pounding heel strikes. The most common issue with regard to form running on a treadmill is the tendency of the machine to almost catch your feet and throw them back under your body with excessive force. This can make you stumble, trip up or even fall. Personally, I feel caged on a treadmill; free sprinting is the only way to go!

*Tip- Walking and running outside require you to do all of the work to pull yourself forward. A treadmill's motor pulls the surface along, doing some of the work for you; it's actually equivalent to walking on a slight downgrade. If you do run on a treadmill, compensate by raising the grade at least 1% - this will help your muscles to work just as hard as they would outside on a flat surface. We'll talk more about treadmill grade and intensity in future updates.

## Sprinting with Great Form

Since we're talking about sprinting hill for maximum efficiency and results, let's do a quick rundown of how to get the most out of your sprinting form on a hill or on flat ground. Here are some basic points of good technique to build on!

Sprinting is always done placing the energy and point of contact on the ball of the foot. The spring-like ability of the calf muscles really come into play here and help catapult your body forward with speed and power. Try running fast on your heels. It just can't be done but it sure lends some comic relief when you see it.

Lean forward into your stride when sprinting up hills, especially during the acceleration phase of the sprint. This increases power output and helps you drive up the hill.

When on flat ground, make it a tall posture. Run erect, with full extension of the back, hips and legs as opposed to a squatty posture. You'll get more out of each stride (again, lean forward while sprinting up hills.)

Relax. This means moving with ease as opposed to struggling hard to move. Let the whole act of the sprint flow. Hands not clenched, open and fingers loose. Each step should be efficient and rhythmic, just like a rep of barbell curls!

Drive. This translates to push or power from the extended rear leg, rear elbow drive with a high forward knee drive to make a strike and claw foot action just behind your body's center of gravity.

Drive the arms with each step, keeping them close to your sides (never across the body) elbows at 90 degrees and slightly straightening them as you drive them down to coordinate with the touchdown of the next stride.

## Build it up

I want to remind you of the importance of starting slow and adding more volume/intensity to your sprinting program as you go. If you're overweight or out of shape when you start, don't jump right into it hard-charging. That's great but ease into the challenge. You'll be less likely lose motivation and fall out or quit. Worst-case scenario would result in injury so avoid this at all costs. The soreness you may feel will be bad enough so just make sure you take it easy and be patient with yourself!

## Superset Sprints- a secret weapon for results

If you hadn't guessed by now, I'm big on hill sprints and I'm big on weight training. Why not combine the two for a short but amazing session that carves your body into a walking anatomy chart? Doing hill-sprint supersets with weights will do just that. The whole idea of a super set is to combine two exercises or movements back to back non-stop for one big set that is more challenging and usually, more painful. Why do I do this? Because I'm a masochist? I don't think so but what I do think is the "good pain" of making amazing results is addictive and crashing through these little pain barriers to get there cranks up your results that much faster. That part of it is not just for superficial endeavors but moreover it's for training your mind to keep going no matter what the struggle or barrier. This sort of mental training can be applied to anything else in your life and I have found it to be a great tool when things get painful in other areas of life.

Ok, my superset training has given my clients and myself results beyond my wildest dreams. If I told people my training techniques were going to put me on the cover of Men's Fitness magazine back in the day, they would have told me to keep dreaming and that's just what I did along with train with the following methods!

The following is an example of a hill sprint superset routine I employ as my cardio 2-3 times per week with amazing results in under 40 minutes and it keeps me shredded!

Bring a pair of dumbbells or kettle bells with you. Start with a warm-up of a light run or a brisk walk up the hill a couple of times. The first sprint up the hill, make it 50% effort of whatever feels close. Remember to always stretch between sets!

- *Set 1- Sprint up the hill at (or what feels like) 50% effort. Walk back down. Once at the bottom, immediately perform a set of push-ups at a fast pace with perfect form, going close to failure. This usually means your pace is coming to a fast halt.*
- *Set 2- Sprint up the hill at over 50% effort; walk back down. Immediately do a set of bent-over rows with the dumbbells then a 2nd set of pushups.*
- *Set 3- Sprint up the hill at over 75% effort. Once at the top, drop and do a set of crunches until you feel a good healthy burn in them. Walk back down. Immediately do a set of bent-over rows.*
- *Set 4- Sprint up the hill at close to 100% effort; once at the top, drop and do a set of straight leg lifts, walk to the bottom- another superset a set of pushups and bent-over rows.*
- *Set 5- Sprint up at near top effort again, once at the top drop and do a set of diamond pushups followed by*

*a set of crunches. Walk back down, once at the bottom, do a set of bent-over rows/pushups.*

- *Set 6- Deep-walk lunge to the top this set, alternating each leg to the top. Once up there, do a set of crunches followed by a set of body-weight squats. Burn baby, burn! Walk back down, do another superset of pushups and bent-over rows.*

- *Sets 7-12- Just perform sprints at tolerable levels of effort, but shooting for 75% or above. Don't know what that is or how to identify it? Don't worry if you're sucking major 02 you're right where you need to be in terms of body fat loss. You'll quickly learn to recognize what these levels are and how to feel and listen to your body. It just takes time but all the best athletes in the world share this trait. You will too. Keep rest minimal, no more than 60 seconds; shoot for 30-45. Let's talk about some other options:*

## The rest-reduction superset

What I mean here is instead of building up your effort percentage sprinting up the hill, keep that relatively equal each set but reduce the rest time between each sprint. What you have is more intense sets just from forcing your body to keep up with the ever-increasing pace. The session would resemble something similar to this:

- *Set 1- A warm up, 50% effort going up. Back down, stretch for a couple minutes, rest time around 3 minutes.*
- *Set 2- Pace increased, more of a sprint up the hill close to 75% effort- a quick paced run up the hill but not an all-out sprint. Reduce the rest time by 30 seconds.*

- *Set 3- Same 75% effort up the hill. Jog it back down, reduce the rest time by another 30 seconds, you're down to 2 minutes.*
- *Set 4- You get the idea. By the time you are done, the rest time is gone and you hit the bottom and immediately go back up for another sprint. If you're able to knock a few of these out, congratulations! Your conditioning is awesome and I'd be willing to bet your body fat percentage in on the decrease as well! This scheme is almost harder than increasing the effort up the hill- it's time-based more than effort-based so shoot for around 20 minutes nonstop. You be the judge and try both methods.*

## Body-squat supersets

This method is best used for flat-ground sprints, as the body-weight squats act as an alternate for the hills. When you are up for it, go ahead and try the squats on the hill sprints. But, I prefer to keep the movements for upper body on hill sprint days. Why? My legs are fried enough taking on the resistance that the hill offers. This type of training is an all-out assault on body fat stores. Squats are arguably the best movement to perform in terms of fat loss, HGH release plus strength and conditioning so when you superset them with 50 yard sprints you can begin to understand how this will melt fat off of your body like a lit wick on a candle. It is important to always stretch between sets and since you hit a set of squats between sprint reps, keep the sprints under an all-out effort. You can better pace yourself this way and sense your fatigue levels much better. Hey, you are doing two tough activities back to back; it doesn't matter if you are using zero weight on the squats. Your lungs and legs are already working overtime to propel you through the sprints. If you are already a strong sprinter and have a lot of experience squatting with great form, then feel free to bring some hand held weights out to the field for more of a challenge. Just make sure you know your limits and don't over train! Take 60-90 seconds between sets stretching and catching some O2.

## Simple Intervals

Hardly "simple" because they work and hurt like hell, this method is one that can be practiced on a treadmill or track much easier. Remember to always warm up to protect your body from injury, get the blood flowing and primed for amazing results. Have a stopwatch ready if you're outside.

Traditional Sprints (Outdoor on Track)

## The warm-up:

- *2-minute brisk walk right into a 25% easy jog (40 seconds)*
- *2-minute brisk walk right into a 50% run for (30 seconds)*
- *2-minute brisk walk right into a 90% sprint (15-20 seconds)*
- *Finish the warmup with a 3-4 minute easy walk.*

## The session:

Sprint at 100% effort or your very best (5 to 10 sec) then walk briskly for 4 minutes. Repeat this for sets- however many you can do before you feel a good fatigue setting in but shoot for about 20 minutes! Throw the old notion of running on a dreadmill for an hour at a time out the window! Remember to listen to your body! Cool down afterward and stretch.

# Incline Walking (Treadmill)

## The warmup:

5 min walk (flat, zero grade) then fast walk (incline grade) bump it up to a brisk pace at the 2:50 mark. Get an additional few minutes walking at the elevated heart rate.

## The session:

The PEAKS: Very brisk walk at the highest incline that can be sustained for 30 to 60 seconds. For the first half of this session keep the brisk walk well away from running. For the last half of the session, inch ever-so-closer to having to run at that incline. Gauge the incline to suite your fitness. This is very much like a pyramid set, so gauge the incline according to your fitness level. This however, is NOT a pass to avoid challenging yourself. Keep the incline at the highest and tweak it from there.

*Tip- Like sprinting, walk on your toes. This activates your calves more effectively!

The VALLEYS: 4 min walks. Again, the name of the game here is INTENSITY. Keep it challenging, so reduce the incline and pace by third's. If you're winded (you should be) and it's not enough then cut the resistance/pace in half. I want you to listen to your body; be instinctive and go by feel. Always strive to challenge yourself and make it difficult but allow yourself to keep the pace at the same time. If you do the peaks right, the valleys will be a relief but also a challenge in their own right. Don't cheat yourself!

## Stairs (multiple flights or stadium steps)

### The warmup:

A quick, 2 minute walk on flat ground then walk up the flight of stairs or the top of the stadium. Walk back down to the starting point. Follow that with an easy jog up the steps. Walk down the steps, follow that with a 2 minute brisk walk then run up steps. Walk down at get 3 minute brisk walk. Get ready for results!

### The session:

This mode of training on stairs is almost (if not more) effective than sprinting hills. You can tell by the burning sensation it puts your legs and lungs through. You be the judge!

Sprint up the flight of stairs, always sprinting on the toes! This will utilize the calves and give you a much more springy, powerful step. Walk back down the steps, immediately get 4 minute walk

Repeat these sets until you recognize your body telling you it's getting taxed or go for around 20 minutes- that's it! Preferably, don't train stairs on weight-training days; due to the intense nature of the previous training modes don't perform them more than 3x per week.

*Tip- If the stairs you're on are too short, double up on them and give the sprints a bigger ROM! (by now you know that's Range of Motion)

## Fifties

This style of hill sprint training is more like an interval set up without the track. All it means is every other sprint you perform, interval a 50% swing in effort. After a couple warm up reps, begin set one with a 50% effort up the hill. Set two bring it close to 100% effort. Set three back down to 50%, set four 100%. It really gives you a chance to hang on to some glycogen in those legs a little longer and lets your lungs recover as well. You're able to go a little longer. Just don't forget to bring a stopwatch to keep track of your rest time between reps! Shorter time for the 50%'s and an extra 30 seconds or so for the 100's! The total session should last only between 20 and 30 minutes, no more if you do it right.

# CHAPTER 5: The Fuel – Eat for Ultimate Results!

Turning back the clock on aging doesn't just happen by pushing weights and sprinting up hills- although those are huge factors in your success. As a matter of fact that's only part of the Ultimate Body equation. As I'm sure you already know eating healthy isn't always easy. From work lunches, to tight schedules, to kids to a lack of time to prepare or even learn about how to make better choices it seems the odds are stacked against us when it comes to eating for your most ultimate shape ever. What you need to know is that A) It's easier, cheaper and more basic than you think to make healthy food choices, and B) Healthy food choices can and do taste great. Besides training properly, what we put inside our bodies is a crucial factor in holding back the natural progression of aging that we all experience. We have a choice to adapt and improve. We can either let daily life and stress sway us to make the wrong choices, feel tired, get fat, then feel more tired or just plain give up as we age. This does not have to happen as we all have to power within ourselves to fuel our bodies with the right stuff to actually slow the aging process to a standstill. Like I've said numerous times if you can use a can opener and boil water, you know how to prepare a great tasting, healthy meal that fuels the Ultimate Body prescription!

# *Terms and methods to apply*

**Amino Acids-** The building blocks of the proteins that you put in your body and what your muscles are comprised of. There are twenty-two standard amino acids of which eight of them are called essential and must be obtained through nutritional intake.

**Arginine-** This one has been big lately; overhyped with so many nitric oxide (N.O.) products floating around in the supplement world these days. Many of these products boast a "secret" to achieving a ripped, muscular physique. Just be aware and read the labels! It is a non-essential amino acid as your body can produce it most of the time but still can be delivered through food sources including some dairy products vegetable sources like granola and certain types of nuts.

**Antioxidants-** Molecules that can slow or prevent the breakdown or oxidation of other molecules. Oxidation produces compounds called free radicals that begin the process of breaking down our cells. Many foods that combat this horrible process are readily available to us and you will know about them! Just like your training, antioxidants will also slow the aging process considerably.

**Calorie-** The basic unit of measurement of food energy that is available through cellular respiration. I'm sure you've heard of good and bad calorie sources when it comes to your food choices. We are going break it down in an easy-to-understand method for ultimate results.

**Carbohydrate-** A great source of energy for the body. They contain carbon, hydrogen and oxygen. Yes, there are good and bad ones to consume as far as your health and shape are concerned, types include starches, sugars and fibers. They contain four calories per gram and contain a sufficient amount of water (hence the "hydrate" part) close to three grams per one of carbohydrate. This is why those misleading "low carb" restrictive diets will work so quickly by simply losing water weight, not fat. Just like the weight is lost, it comes back just as fast and more of it. Those diets work for some but not so well for the majority that try them. It's just not a realistic way to eat day by day.

**Cholesterol-** Types of fats that historically got a bad rap. There really is only one "bad" type, the LDL (low density lipoprotein) and the HDL (high density lipoprotein) being the good. LDL is responsible for much of the artery clogging and heart disease going on these days but can be controlled and reduced through proper nutrition exercise and in some cases medication. The HDL is plays a vital role in the production of many hormones in the body.

**Essential fatty acids (EFAs)-** Much like the essential amino acids, these are good fats our bodies can't produce on their own so we must get them from food sources including safflower and flaxseed oil. They important for cellular health and hormone production, which helps us achieve optimal shape!

**Fats-** We can all picture this word. But not all fat is bad. There are two types, saturated (the bad) and unsaturated (the good). Fat has the most calories of all the macronutrients at nine calories per gram. Unsaturated fat is broken down into two types, monounsaturated and polyunsaturated. More on fat's details in a bit.

**Fructose-** A type of sugar that comes from various fruits. It's a white solid that is the most water-soluble of all the sugars. It's found in honey, tree fruits and some root vegetables. It's derived from the digestion of table sugar (sucrose)

**Glucose-** A simple sugar and important carbohydrate in biology. Cells use it for energy as it's the main sugar found in our blood.

**Glycogen-** The main source of stored carbohydrate energy found in our muscles. It is made primarily by the liver. During intense anaerobic training (weight training) your body taps into the muscles for glycogen and when it's depleted you feel flat and tired- you can tell when you're done. When in your muscles, they look and feel much more dense and full.

**Glycemic Index-** A scale to measure the effects of different carbohydrates on our blood sugar levels. A 0-100 ranking is given to rank each food's response to glucose. Foods below 50-60 on the scale are considered low GI and those above are considered high GI.

**Linoleic acid-** One of the essential unsaturated fatty acids. More precisely an omega-6 poly-unsaturated fatty acid. It must be taken in from our meals and without it, things like poor wound healing and dry hair and skin can occur. It's found primarily in safflower and grape seed oil. You may have heard of the supplement CLA (conjugated linoleic acid) This supplement is said to effectively target the breakdown of belly fat and offer a whole host of other benefits. It's man-made from plant oils and not the natural source found in ruminant animals which is always the better way in the long run.

**Linolenic acid-** Another essential fatty acid. This one is found mainly in flaxseed oil; it is an omega-3 poly-unsaturated fatty acid and one that helps the body metabolize fat and achieve ultimate results. See? Some fats you must have.

**Macronutrients-** The class of chemical compounds that we as humans consume for energy and growth in larger amounts. They include carbohydrates, fats and proteins.

**Micronutrients-** All other nutrients needed throughout life but in small quantities. These include vitamins such as A or C and minerals (referred to as microminerals) such as chromium or zinc.

**Metabolism-** The burning of food or fuel (hopefully healthy nutrients) in the body. This term is thrown around loosely in the fitness and supplement industries but it means the same thing. We all have different rates or "metabolic rates" at which our bodies burn food we consume for energy. Many factors play a role in what this rate is such as 1) What and how often you eat 2) exercise or caloric consumption 3) muscle mass and body type (from chapter 2.4) Our genetics play a huge role in this term; we can however maximize our genetics and force our bodies to make amazing transformations! Just remember that muscle is a metabolic engine and you must fuel it, train it and preserve it at all costs. In turn, starve the fat. This is simply achieved by training with the principles in this eBook and making the right food choices. When you do this, you are going to tire of the number of times people approach you with questions about how you got your Abs to show up!

**Protein-** Primarily what our muscles, enzymes and some hormones are comprised of. Built of amino acids and essential for growth of lean muscle to help burn off unwanted belly fat, one gram of protein contains four calories. Animal proteins contain the essential amino acids and those from vegetable sources contain a few. Once ingested in a meal, proteins are broken up into amino acids and sent to repair and grow your new fat-burning muscle tissue!

**Saturated fats-** Historically referred to as the "bad fats" that should be avoided if at all possible, yet as of late that is just not the case. Comprised of a carbon backbone, these fats have zero open links in that backbone. There are good ones however- from natural sources like organic animal fats, coconut and palm oils. Our brains are made up mainly of cholesterol and saturated fats. If you skimp on these essential fats, you also could be skimping on your brains ability to function optimally; not to mention that these good fats help us shed unwanted fat off of your body! The bad ones are the processed saturated fats that preserve shelf life of processed food. Not a good thing to be putting in your stomach because it will reduce your shelf life!

**Unsaturated fats-** "Good" fats by most standards. Also having a carbon backbone, unsaturated fats have open links in theirs. Mainly coming from plant origins, this type of fat includes the healthy linoleic and linolenic types found safflower, sunflower and flaxseed oils. I put mine in my morning bowl of oatmeal, and I can't even taste it.

**Thermogenic-** A.k.a fat burners, referring to a type of supplement that increases body temperature and thus supposedly increases caloric consumption. Depending upon if they are summoned through intentional movement of the muscles, thermogenics "thermos" can be classified as one of the following: 1)Exercise associated thermogenesis (EAT) 2)Non-exercise associated thermogenesis (NEAT) 3) Diet induced thermogenesis (DIT)
Most of these formulations include the basic ingredients and it seems more are being found to produce similar effects on a daily basis. These basic ingredients are caffeine, ephedra, (alkaloids) bitter orange, ginger root, guarana or the like. Just make sure you read the labels and

again, read the labels as some of these products pack a punch that's not suitable for people that aren't used to them or higher intensity training- sometimes that combo can make you sick. Always safe to get your Doctor's take!

**Supplement-** A term referring to a pill, powder or tablet containing one or a combination of nutrients, vitamins or sometimes who knows what. The supplement industry has turned into a multi-million dollar machine. While not all supplements are useless money-wasters, some of them are. Ones I believe in are various protein powders, creatine, glutamine and some thermogenics. Just keep in mind that supplements do just that. They supplement a pre-existing healthy diet and exercise routine and are NOT meant to take its place. Now there are some meal-replacement shakes containing carbohydrates and proteins to serve as a meal stand-in but they could never take the place of real, solid food. Use them wisely, like a between meal snack you'll see in the week meal plan example I've included. An important note about supplements- mostly of the "fat burning" lot is that they are not regulated by any governing body such as the FDA so tracking exactly what is in some of these mysterious pills is a murky business. What you have to keep in mind is this: The next time you check the ingredients on a supplement bottle, you will probably see a "proprietary" blend on the label. This is the supplement company's way of not telling you what and how much is actually in the stuff. It should make you raise an eyebrow and it's legal. Just make sure you do your research before taking anything. Read reviews. Your health is the true wealth.

## *READ THE LABEL BEFORE YOU BUY IT*

By law, foods must have nutritional content labels on them to be sold- even the "healthy" foods so you better know how to read them! These days, countless products lining grocery store shelves and their bold artwork appeal to everyone. Food that claims to be low in fat and cholesterol-free calls out to the health-conscious consumer. Turn a can or box around and you'll discover the back or side covered with nutritional values, a listing of ingredients and other food label information. For me, it's a really simple process. If the food is processed, I stay away. The less ingredients the better. The three big buttons the processed food industry loves to push on consumers are the most unhealthy and addictive: Sweet, salt and fat. So many items containing shelf-life increasing crap will sabotage your efforts in the gym and more importantly could make you sick with any number of ailments down the road.

Research has shown that eating a well-balanced, nutritious diet reduces the risk of diabetes, coronary heart disease, strokes, some cancers, and osteoporosis. To determine if your family's diet is well balanced, nutritious, and low in fat and cholesterol, you need to look at the nutritional values of the food you're buying, understand what ingredients the food contains, and keep an eye on your child's caloric intake.

Food labels provide these nutritional answers. In addition, labels allow you to comparison shop and make informed food choices. By reading labels, you can feed your family a variety of foods that meets their various nutritional needs.

## Why Food Labels Were Created

Around a century or so ago, food labels barely identified a container's content, but then again then there weren't all these processed food additives causing cancer, diabetes and obesity we have now. Not only were buyers uncertain what ingredients were used to make a product, but quality was still under suspicion.

In the early 1900s, the Federal Food and Drug Act authorized the federal government to regulate the safety and quality of food. Soon the Food and Drug Administration (FDA) required that ingredients be listed. By 1924 the FDA condemned false claims and misleading statements on food labels. Thereafter, the net weight and names and addresses of the manufacturer or distributor had to be stated on labels as well.

In addition to these regulations, a system for identifying nutritional quality in foods was being established. By 1973 nutritional values that supplied information about the amounts of vitamins and minerals had to be listed.

Fast forward to 1990, when the Nutrition Labeling and Education Act called for a major overhaul of food labels. The FDA and the U.S. Department of Agriculture (USDA) made changes to the labels that would make healthy eating easier. The new labels were launched in 1994 and included five important changes:

1. Nutrition information in bigger, more readable type is required for almost all packaged foods. The information appears on the back or side of packaging under the title "Nutrition Facts." The information is also displayed in grocery stores near fresh foods, like fruits, vegetables and fish.

2. A new column of information "% Daily Value" tells people how the food may fit into a healthy diet.

3. The label must include information about saturated fat, trans fat, cholesterol, fiber, sugar, calories from fat and other important information.

4. Serving sizes are now closer to the amount that people actually eat.

5. Health claims such as "light" or "low fat" must meet strict government guidelines so that they are accurate and consistent from one food to another.

## Learning Label Language

At a glance, it may appear as though everything on the shelves either adds fiber to your diet or reduces fat intake. Nutritional information you need to understand to make an informed food choice includes food label claims, calorie requirements, serving sizes, percent daily values, minerals and vitamins, nutrients and fat percentage.

It's important to remember that the information found on food labels is based on an average diet of 2,000 calories per day, although sadly many folks take in many times this amount. Actual caloric and nutritional requirements vary by age, weight, gender, and activity levels. Use food labels as a guide to determine whether a food is generally nutritious, but don't worry so much about exact amounts and stay active!

## Food Label Claims

A food claim is often made by the manufacturer on the front of the package. For example, "fat free" or "no cholesterol." Many people wonder if these claims are for real, as they should. In fact the FDA only allows claims on labels that are supported by scientific evidence.

But even though claims that indicate lower cholesterol, lower sodium, or lower fat content are regulated you still need to be cautious when reading them because most of the time they are not healthy alternatives. The sugar or salt content of some of these products is off the chart. A good rule of thumb is that if humans made it and it has more than 10 ingredients, throw it back on the shelf. It's not going to do your waistline or health any good.

- *Reduced fat has 25% less fat than the same regular brand.*
- *Light means the product has 50% less fat than the same regular product.*
- *Low fat means a product has less than 3 grams of fat per serving.*

Food companies may also make claims such as no cholesterol (meaning there is no animal fat used in making the product), but that does not necessarily mean the product is really low in fat. Just make sure you read the label!

## Serving Size and Servings Per Container

This one gets a lot of people. At the top of each food label you'll see a serving size amount. The serving size is the amount of food a person would need to eat to get the amount of listed nutrients. If you don't read the label and decide to eat the entire package of whatever the food is, you could end up getting 2-3 times more than one serving size. This is a problem. Read, read, READ the labels!

## Food labels and your family

As a parent, you can use food labels to your advantage by using them to plan nutritious and healthy meals for your children (or your parents). The following tips will help you create healthy food choices using food labels. Now is the time to get your loved ones on the right track nutritionally. Try to stay away from processed foods! Start smart habits now! They will thank you for it later down the road. You will be giving them a foundation for a longer, healthy life.

Offer your family a variety of foods. Insufficient amounts of nutrients can lead to malnutrition and open the door to illness. By showing them a variety of healthy foods like plenty of grain products, vegetables, and fruits you can ensure that they take in a wide variety of nutrients to help avoid trips to the Doctor. Choose a diet low in total fat, saturated fat, trans fat and cholesterol. Limit total fat intake to no more than 30% of total calories per day.

Read serving size information. What looks like a small package of food can actually contain more than one serving due to calorie content!

Consume sugar and sodium in moderation; all an adult really needs is a teaspoon a day! Kids need much less. Most products have more than enough salt to last a few meals in one serving. Check the label!

Choose healthy, natural snacks. Those such as potato chips and cheese puffs are high in calories, sodium, cholesterol and fat- all the stuff that makes us fat. Not only that they are low in vitamins and minerals. Healthy snacks should include fruits, vegetables, and whole-grains. These types of snacks will help you lose stubborn belly/body fat and also have a secret fat-burning weapon: fiber. This will help fill you up much quicker without the extra calories. I have all these foods listed for you in this chapter.

Be skeptical of "low-fat" processed foods. This is just a ploy by the countless food companies out there catering to the over-hyped weight-loss market. Good for them but don't fall for it. If the fat has been eliminated or cut back the amount of sugar in the food may have increased. Many low-fat foods have more calories as their full-fat versions in the form of belly-fat producing sugar. If you're going to buy this type of food you are better off buying "low sugar" items but again your best bet is to stay away!

Let's take a look at a typical label:

# Nutrition Facts

Serving Size 4 oz. (113g)
Servings Per Container 4

**Amount Per Serving**

**Calories** 280      Calories from Fat 130

|  | % Daily Value* |
|---|---|
| **Total Fat** 14g | 22% |
| Saturated Fat 3.5g | 18% |
| Trans Fat 2.5g | |
| **Cholesterol** 120mg | 40% |
| **Sodium** 640mg | 27% |
| **Total Carbohydrate** 13g | 4% |
| Dietary Fiber 1g | 4% |
| Sugars 0g | |
| **Protein** 24g | |

| Vitamin A 2% | • | Vitamin C 2% |
|---|---|---|
| Calcium 2% | • | Iron 6% |

*Percent Daily Values are based on a 2,000 calorie diet. Your daily values may be higher or lower depending on your calorie needs:

| | Calories | 2,000 | 2,500 |
|---|---|---|---|
| Total Fat | Less Than | 65g | 80g |
| Saturated Fat | Less Than | 20g | 25g |
| Cholesterol | Less Than | 300mg | 300 mg |
| Sodium | Less Than | 2,400mg | 2,400mg |
| Total Carbohydrate | | 300g | 375g |
| Dietary Fiber | | 25g | 30g |

Calories per gram:
     Fat 9  •  Carbohydrate 4  •  Protein 4

Now let's talk about what we are looking at. If you want, grab your favorite product and follow along as we identify each item.

Starting up at the top, the servings per container or package tells you how many servings are in the whole package. So if one serving is 1 cup and the entire package has 5 cups, there are five servings per package. These quantities are based on the amount people generally eat and they are determined by the manufacturer. Serving sizes are not necessarily recommended amounts but common ones.

Other nutritional information on the package is based on the listed serving size. So if there are two servings in the package and you eat the entire package, then you must double all of the nutritional amounts listed because those amounts are per serving. Make sure you remember that!

**Sodium**
Sodium is a component of salt and is listed on the Nutrition Facts label in milligrams. Small amounts of sodium are necessary for keeping proper body fluid in balance. Sodium also helps with the transmission of electrical signals through nerves. Too much sodium however can worsen water retention and high blood pressure in people who are sensitive to it. Almost all foods naturally contain small amounts of sodium. Sodium also adds flavor and helps preserve food but processed foods contain _way_ too much sodium- breads, chips and many canned foods. If you want to get your Ultimate body and especially Awesome Abs, then go light on the sodium all the way around. It's far better for your long-term health and your body will lose that subcutaneous layer of water that sodium holds in; you will be leaner just from this tip. The average daily diet contains enough

sodium for an entire week of eating. It comes as no surprise why high blood pressure is so common!

## Total Carbohydrate

This number is listed in grams on the label and combines several types of carbohydrates: dietary fibers, sugars and other carbohydrates. Carbohydrates are either simple (the ones to avoid) or complex (the ones we want). Carbohydrates are the most abundant source of calories on earth. The best sources of complex carbohydrates are whole-grains like couscous or brown rice. Other sources include pastas, fruits and vegetables. Carbohydrates should be a person's primary source of energy, providing 40-50% of total calorie intake per day depending on your energy and activity levels. I can tell you this: If you are on a consistent weight training program you will need your share of complex carbohydrates for energy to get through the training sessions. Our bodies need carbs to grow new muscle and your mind needs them to perform at peak capacity as well! As far as the weight loss supplement industry goes, don' get caught up in the new buzz words for carbs- net carbs, impact carbs or effective carbs. These are invented words that only confuse consumers more. Just stay focused on the complex carb sources I have listed for you in this chapter and you'll be fine.

## Dietary Fiber

Listed under total carbohydrate, dietary fiber itself has no calories and is a necessary part of a healthy diet. As of late the weight loss supplement industry has been labeling fiber as "non impact" which you may have seen. They are just trying to find a way to tell you that fiber has no effect on blood sugar levels. High-fiber diets promote bowel regularity, may help reduce the risk of colon cancer and can help reduce cholesterol levels. The best thing about fiber however is that it is very filling and can have you filling full for a longer period of time- great if you are trying to shed inches and pounds! Eat your fruits and veggies for this effect!

## Sugars

Also listed under total carbohydrate on food labels, sugars are found in most foods. Foods such as whole-grain breads are high in complex carbohydrates and are part of a healthy diet. Fruits contain simple sugars but also contain fiber, water and vitamins which make them a healthy choice too.  How many people do you know who got fat from eating fruit? Right me either. Unhealthy junk foods like candy, cookies and soda on the other hand often have large amounts of added sugars. Although carbohydrates have just 4 calories per gram, the high sugar content in snack foods means the calories can add up quickly and these "empty calories" usually contain zero nutrients the body stores as fat.

## Protein

This listing tells you how much protein is in a single serving of a food and is usually measured in grams. Most of the body including muscles, skin and the immune system is made up of protein. If the body doesn't get enough fat and carbohydrates it can use protein for energy.  This again is why you see so many serious long-distance runners that look frail; their bodies begin to burn what little muscle they have left. Foods high in protein include eggs, milk, meat, poultry, fish, cheese, yogurt, nuts, soybeans and various beans, my favorite being black beans. Protein should make up about 25%-30% of a person's daily calorie intake and if you lift weights, you could possible take in a little more. In this chapter I have listed the best protein sources for you make meals with.

## Vitamins A and C

Vitamin A and vitamin C are two especially important vitamins and that is why they are listed on the Nutrition Facts label. The amount for each vitamin in each serving is measured in percent daily values so if a food has 80% of vitamin C you're getting 80% of the vitamin C you need for the day. It's required that food companies list the amounts of vitamin A and C and if they want to they can also list the amounts of other vitamins. (Cereals often do this.)Vitamin A usually appears first on a food label's list of vitamins and minerals. Vitamin A is important for good eyesight and helps maintain healthy skin. It's found in orange vegetables, such as carrots and squash, and in dark green, leafy vegetables. Vitamin C is found in citrus fruits, other fruits, and some vegetables. The body uses vitamin C to build and maintain connective tissues, heal wounds and fight infections.

## Calcium and Iron

The percentages of these two important minerals are listed here also and measured in percent daily values. Food companies are required to list the amounts of calcium and iron and if they want to, they can also list the amount of other minerals (various cereals do this.)

Calcium has a lot of uses in the body but it is best known for its role in strengthening healthy bones and teeth. Milk and other dairy products like yogurt are excellent calcium sources. Children between the ages of 1 and 3 need around 500 milligrams of calcium per day, while 4- to 8-year-olds need 800 milligrams. The calcium requirement for children from 9 to 18 years jumps up to 1,300 milligrams per day - the equivalent of 4 to 4 1/2 cups (about 1 liter) of milk. It's easy to see why most teens in the United States don't get enough calcium every day, but remember that calcium can also be found in other foods as well including fortified orange juice, yogurt, cheese, and green leafy vegetables.

Iron helps the body produce new, healthy red blood cells. Red blood cells carry oxygen, so it's important to get plenty of iron. Teenage girls and women need extra iron to compensate for iron lost in the blood during menstruation. Red meat is the best source of iron but it is also found in iron-fortified cereals, raisins, and dark green leafy vegetables.

**Calories Per Gram**
These numbers show how many calories are in 1 gram of fat, carbohydrate, and protein. This information must be printed on every Nutrition Facts label for reference.

**Calories**
A calorie is a unit of energy that measures how much energy a food provides to the body. The number given on the food label indicates how many calories are in one serving.

**Calories from fat**
The second number, calories from fat, tells the total number of calories in one serving that comes from fat. The label lists fat so that people can monitor the amount of fat in their diets. Dietitians generally recommend that no more than 30% of calories come from fat over the course of the day. That means if the food you eat over

the course of a day contains 2,000 calories total, no more than 600 of these calories should come from fat- but don't be afraid of all fat! Some of them are good and we are going to discuss which ones in this chapter and where to get them.

## Percent Daily Values

Percent daily values are listed in the right-hand column in percentages, and they tell how much of a certain nutrient a person will get from eating one serving of that food. Ideally, the daily goal is to eat 100% of each of those nutrients. If a serving of a food has 18% protein, then that food is providing 18% of your daily protein needs if you eat 2,000 calories per day.

Percent daily value is most useful for determining whether a food is high or low in certain nutrients. If a food has 5% or less of a nutrient, it is considered to be low in that nutrient. A food is considered a good source of a nutrient if the percentage is between 10% and 19%. If the food has more than 20% of the percent daily value, it is considered high in that nutrient.

## Total Fat

This number indicates how much fat is in a single serving of food and is usually measured in grams. Although eating too much fat can lead to obesity and related health problems, our bodies do need some fat every day. Fats are an important source of energy; they contain twice as much energy per gram as carbohydrate or protein. Fats provide insulation and cushioning for the skin, bones, and internal organs. Fat also carries and helps store certain vitamins (A, D, E, and K). But because eating too much fat can contribute to health problems, including heart disease, adults and children older than age 2 should have no more than 30% of their daily calorie intake come from fat.

**Saturated Fat and Trans Fat**
The amount of saturated fat appears beneath total fat. In 2006, manufacturers were required by the FDA to list trans fats separately on the label and for good reason.

Saturated fats and trans fats are often called "bad fats" because they raise cholesterol and increase a person's risk for developing heart disease. Obviously, this holds truth. Both saturated and trans fats are solid at room temperature (picture them clogging up arteries!). Saturated fat usually comes from animal products like butter, cheese, whole milk, ice cream, and meats. Some trans fats are naturally found in these foods too; they're not all bad. But they are also in vegetable oils that have been specially treated, or hydrogenated so they are solid at room temperature like the fats in stick margarine or Crisco®, for example. Other foods that may contain trans fat include some cookies, crackers, fried foods, snack foods and processed foods. These are the ones you need to stay away from at all costs, more on these later.

If the label does not list trans fat, look in the ingredient list for words such as "hydrogenated," "partially hydrogenated," or "shortening" to tip you off on whether the food contains trans fats.

It's recommended that saturated fats account for less than 10% of daily calorie intake. Trans fat intake should be as low as possible, or non-existent. The stuff is that bad.

## Saturated Fat

Unsaturated fats are also listed under total fat. These are fats that are liquid at room temperature. Foods high in unsaturated fat are vegetable oils, nuts and fish. Unsaturated fats are often called "good fats" because they don't raise cholesterol levels like saturated fats do.

## Cholesterol

Cholesterol is listed under the fat information - it's usually measured in milligrams. It's important in producing vitamin D, some hormones and in building many other important substances in the body. Cholesterol can however become a problem if the amount in the blood is too high. This can increase the risk of developing atherosclerosis, a blockage and hardening of arteries that can lead to a heart attack or stroke later in life.

Most of the cholesterol that a person needs is manufactured by the liver. However, dietary sources such as meat and poultry, eggs, and whole-milk dairy products, also contribute to a person's cholesterol level.

The bottom line is always read all the labels on the foods you normally buy and use your new food label savvy to create a well-balanced diet. It may seem complicated at first but by using food label information to select foods that are high in nutrients, in a little time you will make better food choices automatically. Buying a variety of foods will go a long way in meeting your nutritional needs and achieve that Ultimate Body you're looking for. When you see your body changing you simply won't want to put anything else in it.

## *Protein sources for the "Pros"*

*When we are talking ground chicken or turkey, make sure you buy BREAST meat. It will say on the package if it is. If it is not breast meat, you are getting a lower quality meat higher in fat calories- and who knows what else. There has also been a lot of buzz about organic or "free range" meats. As you have probably heard, factory/farm raised animals are said to be pumped full of hormones, antibiotics and salt solutions to plump them up and genetically alter them for growth. I don't know about you but I don't want those harmful industrial chemicals in my meat. So, for the most part I think a solution could be to only eat organic, natural or "free range" meats. The touchy part here is those terms are used very loosely, meaning "free range" referring to animals raised for meat the U.S. Department of Agriculture stipulates that free-range chickens have access to the outdoors and free-range cows and sheep must be "grass fed" and live on a range. No other criteria such as the size of the "range", the amount of space individual animals must have or care and handling are required so you be the judge. It's interesting, growing up I don't think we had anything close to what is now called organic or free range meats, there were just far less hormones and antibiotics used on meat at that time and for all practical purposes the two are the same thing. These days the terms seem more like a marketing ploy but if it means less chemicals; reverting back to a time when there were more "ranges" (cow pastures) then I'm all for it. "Natural" meats supposedly contain no artificial ingredients and are only minimally processed. Animals raised for natural meats are not fed hormones or antibiotics although they may be fed corn and other grains that have been treated with pesticides. Now for the big one, "organic." Sure sounds wholesome, doesn't it? In order for meat products to be certified organic, farmland must be free of synthetic herbicides, pesticides and fungicides for at least three years. After that the land can then be used to grow crops used for a pasture or feed for farm animals. The animals are not treated with any chemicals or growth hormones and must be fed 100% certified organic feed. They too must have access to roam free on the "range". Growing up in rural Texas I have eaten my share of red meat and poultry, most of which has not been organic or anything of the sort and my health hasn't been better than it is now.  As far as taste goes I couldn't tell you I sense a huge difference except maybe the psychological one. Currently the prices for these types of foods are a bit higher but as demand grows the prices should come down.

Look for the following at your store or market. My fridge is always stocked with these:

Chicken breast (canned, ground, tenders) turkey breast (ground or cutlets) tenders, ostrich, buffalo, egg whites, whole eggs or egg beaters, swordfish, orange roughy, haddock, salmon, tuna, crab, lobster, shrimp, scallops, lean ham, low fat cottage cheese, soy beans, lean ground beef, top round steak, flank and top sirloin steak are all great fat-burning protein sources. For a meal all you need is a portion the size of your fist, no larger. Grill, broil, sear, bake, boil, stir fry are the approved ways to cook your meat. Never deep fry your meats. In addition to protein, iron and other micronutrient content found in these meats they also contain healthy amounts of fats. Yes, some animal fat is good for us as the ones listed are of a lower fat content.

* Be sure to watch how much shrimp and lobster you take in. They have a higher cholesterol content that other protein sources. For example I only have those items 3-4 times or meals per month.

* Egg yolks are higher in cholesterol as well but I still eat the whole egg. I just limit my intake. There are just too many nutrients in the yolk to pass up, including most of the protein.

* When buying turkey or chicken cuts for sandwiches, always ask for low sodium at the deli. This in itself will have you losing inches on your waist and in your face due to the water loss. I personally never buy the pre-packed meat. See how much salt they put in it and you'll understand why.

## *Carbohydrate sources to stock up on*

Remember, carbohydrates are what our bodies use for energy. Our muscles need them to grow and maintain the fat-burning process. Just make sure you are getting them from the correct sources, COMPLEX. The following includes the types your body can use most effectively for your ultimate body.

Add these to your grocery list:
- *Old-fashioned or steel-cut oat meal*
- *stone-ground, sprouted grain or millet bread*
- *Greek yogurt (also higher in protein)*
- *skim/1% milk*
- *acai berry (can be juice)*
- *apples, oranges, bananas, melons, strawberries*
- *barley*
- *buckwheat pasta*
- *steamed wild rice, steamed brown rice*
- *pumpkin, squash, yams, baked or sweet potato*
- *quinoa and couscous- both of which are also very high in protein for a grain and to me are  super-foods.*

These listed are complex unrefined carbohydrates, which should be distinguished from simple carbohydrates- these are the sugars, which supply dead calories and should be avoided. You can't go wrong with fruit in my book. They are simply a great choice for any snack food or addition to any meal. The antioxidant and fiber content are huge benefits to adding them to your regular menu! They help fill us up, keep us young and give us nutrient-rich choices.

## What about veggies?

Look for these favored vegetables at your market:

- *Broccoli, carrots, asparagus, green beans, spinach, tomato, peas, brussel sprouts, artichoke, cabbage, celery, zucchini, cucumber, mushrooms, onions, cauliflower.*

Keep in mind that these are not typically consumed for their carbohydrate content but more so for their nutrient/fiber/antioxidant content. If you do not include a portion of vegetables in your meal plan a good multi-vitamin could be beneficial but again these are manmade and if you can get your nutrients from natural sources in your foods. I would go that route. Grill, steam, boil, bake and never fry your veggies. In a pinch you can always microwave them.

You may have heard of the "caveman" aka Paleolithic diet. I believe these diets are healthy for the most part and my diet models them in some form here and there. I scale my carbohydrate intake up or down pertaining to how much muscle I am trying to hold on to, gain or lose. You can lose weight on this type of diet but you may feel tired and not have the energy needed to perform intense training sessions due to lack of carbohydrate. It's a great solution for someone who prefers not to be active or workout on a regular basis but you still may feel the effects on your mental state without a steady intake of carbohydrate from healthy sources. We need them to perform at high physical and mental levels.

Salads are a great way to make a super-nutritious, fat burning meal very quickly. Some of my favorite leaves are: Baby spinach, mixed herb salad, romaine and arugula. Get your favorite salad mix, cover it with a favored meat or protein source and put a little couscous on top. To make your own healthy dressing, have these ingredients on hand: Pressed olive oil, vinegar or lemon juice, salt and pepper.

Extras if you wish, herbs, spices, fruit or other low-sodium flavorings. Mustard is a good additive; it actually helps hold your dressing together so it can't separate as easily. The ratio of oil to vinegar should be about 3 to 1. Whisk together in a bowl or shake it up in a shaker. That's it! Enjoy!

## *Fat: The Big Fat Facts*

Ok here we go. The bad word. The food industry and society in general has had a field day with this word, made us fear it, shamed us for eating it and made a ton of cash by selling us bogus "low fat" or "no fat" products and in the process created a ton of confusion about it. It all started back in the late 80's when our Surgeon General warned us to cut back on dietary fat intake due to health consequences. The result was product after product cutting fat out but almost doubling the sugar or bad carbohydrate content. I'm about as sick of it as you are. The take home lesson here is: Don't be afraid of all fat! There are some good fats that you need to actually help your body burn off stubborn body fat! (even saturated!) To begin, a healthy supply of the right kind of dietary fat is vitally important in your over-all health. Fats comprise one of the main components of the cell membranes throughout your entire body. Natural healthy fats play many roles in optimum performance of the human body. For example, did you know that a diet too low in good fats can actually hamper your testosterone production? We know what that means: Less fat-burning muscle on your frame and this means more fat on that same frame! Ladies, no need to fear your testosterone is going to pump your muscles up to manly proportions. Not possible! It will however keep everything in top working order and primed for optimal fat burning capability. We just need to be eating the right kinds of fat. When I hear one of these so called health and nutrition "experts" talk of how you need a diet Absent of dietary fat I have to step in and ask them spot on what kind of fat they are referring. If they say the right ones I let them off the hook. Here is the issue: Any diet or plan that restricts any one of the macronutrients can lead you to problems. As a matter of fact the good fats help you to burn stubborn belly fat off your body! For your Ultimate Body we are about balance and ease, not restrictions (except for the man-made trans fats of course)

Ok, let's get you in the know about which fats to eat and which ones to avoid at ALL costs. Let's first have a look at the different types of fats and what they are.

**Various oils:** Olive oil is approximately 70% monounsaturated and only 16% saturated fat. Always get "extra virgin" which is a much more pure form of olive oil as it comes from the first pressing of olives. The highest antioxidant content olive oil, extra virgin olive oil is not produced with the use of harmful industrial solvents like many other types of olive oils on supermarket shelves (such as highly refined soybean oils.) This is the only oil I use when preparing my salad dressings. A tablespoon a day is a good amount for overall health. Walnut oil has been shown to lower triglycerides which in turn lower the risk for coronary heart disease. Grape seed oil is believed to lower bad cholesterol (LDL) in the arteries. It is great for cooking as it can take higher temperatures than olive oil and has a higher smoke point.

**Avocados or fresh guacamole:** This one can qualify as a super-food in my book. Avocados are high in beta-sitosterol, a compound that has been shown to lower cholesterol levels. Avocados are about 60% monounsaturated and 25% saturated fat. They are an excellent source of glutathione, an antioxidant that shows promise to be important in preventing aging, cancer, and heart disease. One cup of avocado has about 25% of the recommended daily value of folate. Studies show that people who eat diets rich in folate have a much lower incidence of heart disease than those who don't. Avocados are the best fruit source of vitamin E, an essential vitamin that protects against many diseases and helps maintains overall health. Try them in wraps, tops of salads and in sandwiches. When it comes to store-bought guacamole, make certain you read the label. Many have processed additives that won't do a body good. Remember when it comes to buying any food, the less ingredients the better. Keep it naturally healthy and your body will respond amazingly well.

**Tropical oils:** (Coconut oil is my favorite.) This one has countless amazing benefits that include hair care, skin care, maintaining cholesterol levels, weight loss and increased immunity. First, some facts: coconut oil is more than 92% saturated fat. I know that sounds bad but hear me out! The fat in coconut oil is about 65% of what are called medium chain triglycerides (MCTs). Of this, about 50% is an

MCT called lauric acid. Our bodies convert lauric acid into monolaurin, which is reported to enhance the immune system. Additionally, MCTs are utilized as an immediate energy source and are NOT stored as body fat. The fat in coconut oil actually helps us lose body fat! The reason behind this being that coconut oil contains less calories than other oils, its fat content is easily converted into energy and it does not lead to accumulation of fat/dangerous plaque in the heart and arteries.

Coconut oil helps in boosting energy and endurance, and enhances the performance of athletes. It is best used as a cooking oil in stir-frying and baking. Also, coconut oil being a healthy saturated fat does not oxidize like other poly-unsaturated oils do when exposed to light or heat- this creates damaging free-radicals which age us and break us down. The best sources of coconut fat are organic coconut milk, fresh coconut or virgin coconut oil. Non-hydrogenated palm oil is another great source of healthy fat-burning fat that is saturated in its composition. Don't be fooled into thinking that these types of fats are bad for us. A large chunk of nutrients on our planet consist of saturated fats that humans have been thriving on them since the beginning of time. It's only until recently that western dietary practices have taken food from its natural healthy state and put it through all sorts of chemical processing and refinement that it becomes unhealthy- all for the sake of money.

**High-fat fish:** Wild salmon and other cold water fish (herring, mackerel, black cod, bluefish) offer a great source of natural omega-3 polyunsaturated fats. Since the middle of the 20th century there has been a large addition of omega-6 polyunsaturated fats such as corn oil and soybean oil in our food composition. The typical western diet is way out of balance having too much omega-6 and not enough omega-3 (somewhere in the neighborhood of 20x more) and this can have damaging effects on the body, for example some omega-6 adds to inflammation and omega-3 reduces it. This can be tied to countless health problems we are currently struggling to deal with. Start taking in your omega-3's! Get them from the above listed fish or from the following vegetarian sources: Various nuts such as walnuts or flax seeds. A healthy amount of high-fat fish is equal to 2-3 servings of salmon per week.

**Nuts:** Just about any type of nut is a great source of healthy, unprocessed fat, proteins and other trace nutrients. Cashews, almonds and macadamias bring great sources of monounsaturated fats and they also offer a good source of protein for a power-packed snack. I actually have a handful of peanuts before an intense training session. The fat keeps me full for the duration and fuels me to help avoid crashing and fatigue. A scoop of your favorite nut butter also does the trick! Again, the same rules apply here. Try to avoid nuts that are cooked in oil or processed in any form so go for raw or dry roasted instead. Although they are healthy they are still calorie rich so keep intake in check! To get the heart-healthy benefits all you need is an ounce per serving. Specifically, the following equal one ounce: 24 almonds, 18 medium cashews, 12 hazelnuts, 8 medium Brazil nuts, 12 macadamia nuts, 35 peanuts, 15 pecan halves and 14 walnut halves (3). Pre-storing nuts into small, single-serving containers or bags can help keep the servings in check. All it takes is a one-ounce serving a day (about a handful) or roughly five ounces per week of a variety of nuts. They are so tasty, it's easy to keep eating them. Just think of them as fuel to help you improve your health and not hinder you from hitting your goal of achieving the Ultimate Body!

**Dark Chocolate:** I'm talking the healthy bittersweet type, which has over 70% cocoa content. The cocoa bean in its natural state has a very high concentration of antioxidants and is what makes this chocolate so healthy. The cocoa butter in the bean is approximately 60% saturated fat (steric acid) 38% monounsaturated fat and 3% polyunsaturated fat. In contrast, most milk chocolates, while delicious are only about 30% cocoa leaving the rest of the ingredients comprised mostly of sugar, corn syrup and other shelf-life increasing garbage. Seek out quality dark chocolate with cocoa content in the range of 70-80%.

It will have very little sugar but still a mildly sweet flavor while still smooth and creamy in texture. Keep in mind this is healthy chocolate and has the natural healthy saturated fat we are looking for but it is still calorie dense. So to get the health benefits, a square or two a day will do the job. Additional benefits of dark chocolate include serotonin, which acts as an anti-depressant. On the weight-loss front it contains theobromine and caffeine which are stimulants to help rev-up your metabolism for fat loss. Now that's a healthy piece of chocolate!

**Various seeds:** Flax, pumpkin, sesame and sunflower are all great sources of natural unprocessed healthy fats. More specifically, flax seeds contain high amounts of omega-3 polyunsaturated fat. Because they are prone to oxidation and free radical production, fresh ground flax seed is a better choice. Try it in yogurt, put it in shakes, cereal or atop a salad. If you have flax oil, get the cold-pressed type. Most comes in a light-proof container as it should and make sure you consume it in a few weeks. Heating it destroys the omega-3 so never use it for cooking! Ok, we've covered the good fats that can actually improve our health and our waistlines. Now, let's go over the ones we should try to avoid.

**Fats to avoid at all cost:** Let me preface this by saying that even healthy fats are calorie rich, so limit the intake!

Here's the word you need scope out on labels and if you see it, throw it back on the shelf- "hydrogenated". What is it? It is a process by which hydrogen gas is forced into the oil at a high pressure. Generally, the more solid the oil, the more hydrogenated it is. Two of the best examples I can think of are Crisco and Margarine. A lot of processed foods use soybean or vegetable oils. This is the artificial trans fat that you have probably heard of. In the 90's, they were figuring out that this stuff could have detrimental health effects; ironic because they were originally produced and thought to be healthier than conventional oils. They are used because they increase shelf life and sadly, a way to make more money at the public health's expense. These are oils that are industrially produced and chemically altered. As if that doesn't sound bad enough, they have even more solvents added to them such as hexane for extraction and a metal catalyst to promote the artificial hydrogenation. They increase LDL or "bad" cholesterol levels and decrease HDL "good" cholesterol. There is also evidence that trans fats bioaccumulate in the body, as the digestive system does not know what to do with them. The result is weight gain and lots of it but that's just what we see on the outside. What it does to our insides is far worse.

Fast forward to the present, where many folks scarf down products that contain these horrible fats that could be slowly killing them or setting them up for any number of disease processes. With people putting garbage like this in their bodies passing it off as food it's no wonder heart disease, cancer and obesity continue to rise. To me, the solution is simple. Back to basics. Prepare our own food. Don't buy over-processed food! Your body's appearance, the way you feel and overall health will drastically improve!

## *Out to eat- how to make better choices*

Going out to eat can be a real challenge if you are watching what you put in your body- especially if you're out with friends. Mix that with the fact that some of those friends are not on the plan to get their ultimate body (now would be a good time to invite them) so peer pressure can be an issue! Don't worry, you can sidestep all of that.

Going out to eat doesn't have to be difficult. Most venues these days will cater to the occasional dieter, hard-core fitness enthusiast and everyone else in between. A few of the following may seem like common sense but usually the most obvious things tempt us into making the wrong choices. When I go out to eat I usually treat it like a cheat or reward day and eat whatever I want. This is easy to do if you're on point each and every day, watching what you eat and preparing your own meals as one dinner out isn't going to sabotage a whole week of healthy eating and training. But if I'm not planning on eating for a cheat day and I want to stay on track, I adhere to the following:

Before anything, just remember that nothing tastes as good as being in your ultimate body feels- this one thought has staved off many temptations and kept me focused on the goal! After all, one or two bites later and your cravings for whatever food are gone. Your stomach just needs to be filled. One or two minutes is all it takes! Ok, onto the tips:

- Choose a place that offers variety in the menu. Most spots will prepare a grilled dish that is normally fried if you just ask. If you're out for an event with pals and didn't choose the venue, check the website before you go.
- If you're new to making healthy choices don't go out to eat on the spur of the moment; see if you can pre-plan your meal

to stay focused and don't EVER worry about being ridiculed for making healthy choices. More often than not, this type of behavior from friends just stems from their own insecurities about being lazy and the fact that you're on track to look better at the beach than they are. Most people hate that notion. Use it to be positive and help them to do the same. If they don't honor it, you know the drill. Chances are they will come around when they notice your body and health improving and envy your example.

- Stay away from places that offer entertainment while eating (judgment call) these types of venues usually have some of the most unhealthy preparation methods in use such as deep-frying and salt/sugar drenched family sized portions. I'm from the south, if I can keep it under control you can too!

- Try to avoid buffets or "all you can eat" spots. These types make it all too easy to lose control and binge-eat.

- Don't ever forget about the salad bar. You can fill up on healthy fibrous salads full of nutrient rich ingredients and stave off the bad stuff. Just remember to keep the dressings healthy as well- vinegar and oil, Italian or balsamic dressings are great choices! Just always ask for them on the side.

- This tip is vital: Load up on healthy stuff before you leave the house like fruit and fibrous snacks like veggies or a cup of couscous. It's sort of like going to the market when you're starving so don't ever do it! You are less likely to load up on poor choices out of sheer hunger.

- Don't touch the bread, chip, or appetizer basket if you can help it. The previous helps deter your cravings like magic. If you already zapped your hunger impulse, your cravings will obviously be less likely to win you over.

- Watch out for restaurants that have a mascot. These are almost always places that skimp on ingredients where the poor menu item choices outnumber the healthy ones.
- When you sit down, this is a pivotal point. Order water right away and slam a glass. This will diminish the initial temptation to eat whatever bottomless pit of free munchies that show up. What we often mistake as hunger is only thirst so take advantage of it!
- Portion size, portion size, portion size! When it comes to ordering, most places offer appetizers that have limited calories vs. the full-fledged entre size. Do we really need all of those calories in one sitting?
- If you do somehow get a full-sized dinner portion in front of you, eat half and take the rest home for a another meal. Your body will thank you in the end and you will be happy knowing there is another meal waiting for you the next day and this means less prep time!
- Appetizers alert: Don't forget it's a kitchen they have back there and "something" can come from anything they have on the menu. Salads, fresh fruit or a veggie plate make a great "appetizer" if you must.
- Be wary of anything that comes with a dipping sauce. If you do end up with something breaded or fried, peel it off. Most of the fat calories reside there.  Use mustard, aioli, BBQ sauce or salsa instead of mayo, tarter or any cream sauce they may give you. When in doubt, ask what's in it!
- Salad toppings and soups- avoid cream soups; instead go for broth-based soups. Avoid salads with fried, breaded, or fatty meat toppings. These will ruin an otherwise healthy salad for you. Like we covered before, ask for the grilled versions of meats! See the following:

- Safe preparation methods for anything you eat when dining out: Grilled, boiled (in water) baked, steamed, broiled, poached, stir-fried, panko-fried, roasted, seared or blackened.
- Know your healthy meats we covered previously and how to prepare them
- Stay away from these methods: Buttery, breaded, buttered, fried, deep-fried, pan-fried, creamed, scalloped, au gratin, a la mode
- Sushi watch: This is a deceptively high-calorie food because of the many ingredients like mayonnaise or heavy sugar in the rice; usually about a tablespoon per cup of rice! This allows it to stick together more easily and if you ever wondered why various sushi rolls taste so good, this is a chief reason! Stay away from tempura (fried) sushi and if you order teriyaki chicken bear in mind that this is a fatty, darker meat and higher in calories- unlike white, leaner breast meat. A better alternative is to ask for sashimi and steamed vegetables if you are in the mood for fish. Go easy on the salty soy sauce by asking for a lighter salt alternative. Most sushi spots have it.
- How you eat is almost as important as what you eat. Eating out is not an event or a time to showcase your competitive eating ability. It's a chance to celebrate friends, family and yourself with a good meal.
- Chew your food thoroughly at around 20x per bite. Take your time chewing and between each bite; concentrate on the conversation not the food. Eat your lowest calorie items first: veggies are a good place to start.
- When your food is half gone, ask yourself "Am I still hungry?" Half the time you will be surprised that the answer is no. Just because it's in front of you doesn't mean you have to consume it. Bag up the rest and take it home for a meal tomorrow.

- Deserts: Be smart about them. You can't ever go wrong with fruit as a healthy, sweet alternative as long as it's not buried in syrup, sugar or whipped topping. (fruit pies or cakes aren't included here)

- Total deprivation won't work in the long-term. The key is finding sensible alternatives that allow you to enjoy deserts a little bit at a time. Remember moderation is golden. You can have controlled amounts of whatever you want here and there. One cookie or scoop of ice cream won't derail your entire effort. Use it as a reward once a week. In the meantime substitute sorbet for ice cream to get the same texture.

- Reward yourself with a "cheat day" once a week. Our taste buds are meant to allow you to enjoy your food and eating is one of life's pleasures. So enjoy yourself! Just do it with sense and moderation. Start with one meal per cheat day- load up on pancakes, waffles, syrup, or eggs Benedict. No limits. Or, let it be lunch with a loaded hamburger, nachos or whatever you want. The rest of your meals should stay with your dietary limits to reach your ultimate shape- at least the first month then you can make a couple meals that day cheat meals. Cheat days are great not just because you get to enjoy yourself and have no limits but you get to see what habits you are leaving behind and the fact is you may not miss those things. After a while of seeing your body change and improve, I doubt you would want to put anything but the healthiest fuel in it for the long term!

## What about fast food?

It can be tough to make smart choices out on the road when you don't have much time to eat. Say for example you're in outside sales and you didn't bring your food with you. What/where do you eat for lunch and stay within the realm of health conscious choices? There are good choices out there in fast food. Here's what I do when in that situation:

- You're better off going to a grocery store and buying a premade meal from the deli or ordering a fresh-made chicken salad or low-sodium turkey sandwich. You'd spend more time sitting in the drive-through line waiting for some fried cancer-sticks and sugar-burgers.

- Some markets also have freshly prepared sushi as well. A sashimi salad or roll will work, just watch the rice content and always go for more greens. Always choose the low-sodium version of soy sauce.

- Many if not all the major fast food chains offer "healthy alternatives" on their menus. Things like low cal grilled chicken sandwiches, wraps and salads. Are they better choices than the regular menu items? They offer less "dead" calories and more useful nutrients, they will do in a pinch but there are better choices still. Some places like Chipotle offer "burrito bowls" the salad versions of the higher calorie burritos minus the rice and tortilla. When I eat there, I ask for less rice and more black beans. The dressing is good there too, fresh made salsa. Surprisingly, the meat is of a higher quality there too even though it was previously owned by McDonald's.

- Be wary. Salad dressings are usually full of sodium and processed ingredients at fast food spots. The buns and tortillas used in fast food restaurants are usually filled with sugar and salt, this goes for the "healthy" menu items as well. They do it for taste and to keep you coming back to spend more. I always ask for corn tortillas, as they are much lower in salt and junk-calories. Visit the websites of these restaurants and look at the nutritional content of these items to see for yourself.

- Limit if not eliminate the extremely high calorie, fat and sugar-loaded coffee drinks. Some of them have more calories, fat, sodium and sugar combined than the fattiest hamburger, no lie. Just because it's a coffee drink does NOT mean it's better for you or less calories. Check the nutritional content of these drinks before you consume them- they can grind your fat-burning efforts to a halt.

- The meat in some fast food chains is usually of a lesser quality, chicken or beef. The 'healthy" wraps or sandwiches usually skimp on the meat by offering darker, fattier meat which is the cheaper part of the animal or worse, sometimes mechanically separated or pressed meat. This is still processed meat and the ingredients are a mystery at best.

- I would avoid the major fast food chains all together if possible but if you can't just cut the bread intake, minimize dressings or get packets of balsamic or vinegar/oil and keep them in your glove box. I make my own and keep it in small bottle in my car. Remember to try to plan and be prepared. Your Ultimate Body is well worth some minor prep time isn't it? Certainly your long-term health is!

We spend more money and take in more empty calories eating out than ever before. The U.S. Department of Agriculture estimates that over 30% of our meals are consumed away from home and that number continues to rise right along with our waistline measurement. Nobody is going to look out for your health but you!

Ok, the bottom line once again is moderation. If you stick to these simple rules you will come out on top every time you dine out. This information is your arsenal to do just that. Use my example if you have to- use dining out as your reward for your hard-earned time and effort sticking to the program. Just remember food is fuel to achieve your ultimate body. It's meant to be enjoyed, yes, but don't let it keep you from the body you know you can have. The more you exercise self control the easier it will become and you will slowly notice the cravings disappear- you're on your way!

## Schedules and meal plan examples made easy.

In this section we are going to cover the basic staple ingredients you need to have in your kitchen and meal plan examples. Your nutritional intake is like your training regimen- your chances of success are far greater if you have some sort of a plan; that plan hinges on what your goals are just like your training. Are you a hard-gainer looking to add bodyweight and gain muscle or are you someone looking to slim down and lose weight? Or somewhere in the middle? Any way you slice it, your body and life will definitely benefit from a steady intake of good, clean nutrients and not junk food filled with empty calories and dangerous chemical shelf-life additives. It's amazing that some people's bodies are so far out of whack from a steady intake of processed food and inactivity, when they apply these simple changes to their diets, they experience an almost immediate improvement in how they feel, look and perform.

### Should you be counting calories?

You certainly don't have to- I've never subscribed to a calorie counting nutritional plan myself. I've always been into simplicity, so I'd rather rely on my instinct while eating and then count my portions.

I know some of you may be much more analytical than myself and need to see the numbers; especially if you are just starting this journey. In this case there is a simple equation you can use to find out just how many calories you need to maintain your current weight. It is, after all very beneficial to know just how many calories are going into your body and from where. Let's talk about it.

First, let's find out what your **basal metabolic rate** is (BMR). This number simply identifies how many calories it takes on a daily basis for your body to maintain basic healthy function or put more simply the number of calories you would burn if you stayed in bed all day just to maintain a current weight.

### *The English BMR Formula is as follows:*

Men: BMR = 66 + (6.23 x weight in lbs) + (12.7 x height in inches) - (6.8 x age (years)
Ladies: BMR = 655 + (4.35 x weight in lbs) + (4.7 x height in inches) - (4.7 x age (years)

Once you calculate your BMR and you know what your specific goals are, you then have the number you need to find out roughly how many calories you should be taking in to gain or lose weight and ultimately get the body you want. We do this by plugging in your BMR into a formula called the Harris Benedict equation. Don't worry, I'm the furthest thing from a math whiz so if I can do this, you surely can.

This equation uses your BMR and then applies an activity factor to determine your total daily energy spent in calories. The only element omitted is muscle/lean body mass. Don't forget leaner bodies burn up more calories around the clock than ones holding more fat. For this reason the more muscular body types will need to under-estimate their daily caloric needs and the more overweight body types will over-estimate theirs. The equation is very accurate but allows you to get a more realistic reading if you employ this.

To find out what your total daily caloric needs are, simply multiply your BMR by the most accurate description of your activity levels below. If you are:

- *Sedentary (exercise very little or none) = BMR x 1.2*
- *Lightly active (light exercise/sports 1-3 days/week) = BMR x 1.375*
- *Moderate active (exercise/sports 3-5 days/week) = BMR x 1.55*
- *Very active (hard exercise/sports 6-7 days a week) = BMR x 1.725*
- *Extra active (intense training/sports 7 days/week ) = BMR x 1.9*

The last two descriptions are similar but try to use the one that best defines your activity levels- intensity or effort are not included but you could probably deduct those would be characteristics of more active lifestyles and can help you to pick the best number. The main factor in this equation is frequency.

Once you know the number of calories needed to maintain your weight, you can easily calculate the number of calories you need to eat in order to gain or lose weight:

## So you want to gain weight? (quality not quantity is key)

If you're a hard gainer and want to gain body weight in the form of fat-burning lean muscle (a good goal for all of us) you need to consume more calories than you burn on a daily basis. One pound of body weight is roughly equal to 3500 calories so consuming an extra 500 calories per day will cause you to gain 1-2 lbs a week on average. Doesn't really sound like much does it? But look at that number over a period of a few months. That's a lot of muscle gained at around 24 lbs! You can scale this number up if you want to gain weight faster but I don't usually recommend this. For optimum health, if you increase your calories to gain weight then (health allowing) gradually increase your calories and level of physical activity in order to maintain or increase your lean body mass. With proper weight training modules this can be accomplished with ease.

## Which types of food are best?

This depends on things like age, metabolism and activity levels but for the most part we should all eat foods from the lists covered in this chapter- why make your body process unnatural and potentially toxic foods? Take our hard-gainer for example. Let's say he's an 18-year old ectomorph (remember that?) His metabolism is naturally cranked up so he can probably get away with eating more simple carbohydrates in the form sugars and junk. The best way to gain quality weight is to increase your intake of quality complex carbohydrates, particularly whole grain ones.

Yes, we are what we eat. Also, legumes and fruits would be wise choices- full of vitamins and nutrients to help speed the rest and recovery processes from intense training. Bagels, larger portions of pasta and rice will do an ectomorph well to gain muscle. As far as protein, it's a good idea to consume 1.5 grams per pound of body weight if you're an ectomorph. If you are on the endomorph side, it would be wise to have 1.5 grams per pound of lean body mass. Too much protein can and will be stored as fat, so get your body fat percentage taken and use the lean body mass number for your protein intake.

In order to gain weight, you will have to eat more calories. You will need to include regular exercise and strength training into your lifestyle in order to prevent gaining too much weight as fat. And, as I mentioned, those extra calories should come mainly from additional complex carbohydrate sources we covered earlier in this chapter for the Ultimate Body and look you're after.

Before you start, set up a realistic goal weight- not too much and not too little. Quality muscle and body composition take time; it will happen and it will last if you do it right. You will also find out that you may be one of those "fast gainers" that have a lot of fast-twitch muscle fiber primed for growth and strength. If you do, congratulations! You have mesomorph-like potential and hitting your goal will take less time.

## What about losing weight?

Simple. Just like gaining weight, it's just a mathematical equation. Burn more calories than you take in each day. Do your quick equations to get your BMR and go from there. I think you will find that when you apply the numbers it can give you realistic goals you can see each day. Can you lose weight just from eating less calories and not exercising? Of course, but here are the problems with that approach. For one, many people that have lost weight or inches by dieting or eating smarter in all probability gain some of the weight (if not all of it) back. The reasons for this are easily identified. 1) Not training your body to build and maintain more fat-burning muscle 2) Making that a consistent lifestyle addition on a weekly if not daily basis. 3) Getting on the diet of the month is usually a short-lived affair. Eating the right foods consistently for the long-term is what allows your body to progress. Make it a commitment to get the body you want! By doing this you give your body no choice but to adapt and improve!

Another thing to remember: You didn't gain excess weight overnight and you shouldn't expect to lose it overnight either. Record a starting goal that you can reach in one month. For example, write down that you want to weigh 5 lbs. less than you currently do in one month. Make it small, realistic and attainable. By doing this, you will continue to set goals, achieve them and crash through barriers. It works, try it and see for yourself!

In addition to training smart and making smart food choices, The following are some tricks to help you ease into better progress and lasting results.

## Start dinner with a salad.

By starting dinner with a healthy soup or salad, you will curb your hunger, which will in turn help you keep portion sizes in check and prevent you from overeating.

## Eat breakfast like a king, lunch like a prince and dinner like a pauper.

If you've heard this line then you are already familiar with tapering your calories down as the day progresses. It works, and it's a way to make sure you don't over-eat. Breakfast is the most important meal of the day (aside from your post-workout meal) Breakfast kick-starts your metabolism into high gear and gives you the energy you need later in the day. If you skimp on your meals, which you should never do, make sure it's not breakfast. Some people don't like to eat in the morning, I get that. Just try to get something though, no matter how small. A cup of Greek yogurt with a tablespoon of oats would suffice.

## No more sugary soft drinks- or their "diet" counterparts.

Take home message- stay away from processed food and drink. For every 20 ounces of your favorite soda you drink, you pack on 250 calories. This is one of the simple carbohydrates and empty caloric fillers that really do nothing for your body except taste good and help you pack away the fat. That's a nice little chunk of calories if you're trying to take in less calories a day in order to lose inches so don't indulge! Be strong and think of what you put in your body- is it going to help you reach your goals? The reason I mention diet soda counterparts is because many times I have noticed that people get to thinking just because they are drinking a diet drink they can skimp on other aspects of nutrition- like have a junk-food calorie dinner or lunch one too many times per week. What's more, there virtually zero nutrients in either version of a soft drink. You're much better off having a low-calorie lemonade or water with a squeeze of lime.

## Drink more water.

And lots of it. Reach for a goal of eight glasses per day. Even if you don't drink up to eight, you're drinking more than usual. If you are going to follow the workouts, then you should be getting at least a gallon a day. I have around 1.5 gallons if not more. If it gets boring, try squeezing some lemon or lime in it or using sugar-free sweeteners. In addition to flushing out the toxins in our bodies, good water intake fills our muscles with water, which is what most of our body consists of. Make them able to work at full capacity! On the hunger front, being properly hydrated also keeps hunger cravings at bay.

To talk precise numbers again, there are approximately 3500 calories in a pound of stored body fat. This means if you create a 3500-calorie deficit through smart food choices, exercise or both (the best choice) you will lose one pound of body weight. Most of this weight being pure body fat. Sounds like a lot, I know but you will be surprised to know how fast it actually comes off when you follow the right methods.

A useful starting guideline for lowering your calorie intake is to slightly reduce daily calorie below your maintenance level (BMR). Get the numbers and customize your caloric intake (BMR) When we are talking effective and lasting weight loss, creating too much of a caloric deficit too quickly (many fad diets come to mind) is not a good thing for a few reasons. Your body activates several "survival responses" which are not ideal for fat loss such as:

1. Your body slows the release of fat-burning enzymes such as hormone sensitive lipase and lipoprotein lipase, an enzyme produced in our fat cells and bound to the walls of capillaries. It breaks down triglycerides into free fatty acids and glycerol, which can enter cells for storage or energy production.
2. The body releases less of the hormone leptin, which sends a signal letting the brain know that you're fed and not starving.
3. It all boils down to this biggest negative: The loss of fat-burning muscle tissue.

Muscle is very metabolically active. It requires more calories just to keep it- much more than fat. So when you deplete calories and carbohydrates with a fad diet, your muscle tissue becomes expendable and is the first to go along with water weight. Losing fast weight is never a good answer, it comes back and usually with reinforcements. There is a better way that works for the long term. Reducing calories by 15-20% below your daily calorie maintenance needs is a useful and safe start. You may increase this depending on your weight loss goals. It may help you to have a calorie-counting handbook, you can find them online or at a bookstore for next to nothing. This way, if you want you can see what food has how many calories in it to get a handle on what you need and don't need per serving. Always read the labels of anything you buy! Especially if it's processed. Soon you this stuff will come natural to you and you won't need to refer to a manual of any kind!

I know many people out there don't care to exercise or even sweat for that matter. But if you really want to change your body, to keep stubborn belly fat off of your body for the long term, then a combination of weight training and smart calorie consumption are going to get you there. Can you just lose weight and not train or exercise at all? Yes, but the effects of creating lean body mass in new muscle is what is going to amp up your metabolism as you age by burning off body fat at a much faster rate and keep it off. As you know, your RMR (resting metabolic rate) will continue to slow as you go on in this game of life. Weight training will help keep it cranked up!

The following are meal weekly meal plans to follow. You already have the preferred protein, carbohydrate and vegetable grocery lists to prepare these so now it's time to fuel up! One thing I ask of you is don't fall into the notion that healthy eating is boring, expensive or time consuming. The fact is all of those are false. The meals I list for you are made with ingredients you can find at the $1 dollar store if you want and overall you end up saving money buying basic ingredients vs. going out to eat or buying processed garbage. Moreover they are so simple to prepare and they provide your body the nutrients it needs for ultimate results! Bottom line: You know exactly what you are putting in your body now!

## Sample daily meal plans

**About the snacks-** If you can't or aren't able to make a shake don't worry about it. Those are there just for you to mix it up when you can. But, it's important to not let yourself get hungry so keep a bag of healthy snacks around you at all times, like trail mix, jacketed foods like fruits or your favorite nuts. These snacks will stabilize your blood sugar levels all day and prevent fatigue and keep your metabolism burning strong. Some protein bars are good choices but remember to read the labels! I stay away from most if not all of them, way too many ingredients even in supposed "healthy" protein bars. Some organic brands are proving to be good however. Look for those instead if you end up purchasing bars.

Start your day with your first big glass of water when you roll out of bed. We get dehydrated over night so refill your body and give it the water it needs to function optimally- first thing in the morning!

### *Monday*
**Breakfast-** One cup of steel-cut oatmeal, one tablespoon of flaxseed oil, a handful of frozen blueberries. Frozen fruit is great on hot oats, it cools it off like ice cubes. I will then mix a scoop of my favorite protein powder in a cup of skim or rice milk and pour over the oats. Wash it down with a glass of water and you're done!

**Mid-Morning Snack-** A handful of trail mix or my favorite nut. Have it with a glass of water.

**Lunch-** Quinoa or couscous scramble- Mix a cooked cup of either with black beans and your favorite protein source- for me it's canned turkey or chicken breast. Throw the mix over a small bed of salad greens for a great meal. I cook this meal in bulk and you can see how I do it here. It's super-fast, delicious, lasts a while and it is awesome for the road.

**Mid-Afternoon Snack-** Banana/peanut butter-chocolate protein shake. Add a cup of ice, 1-2 cups of skim milk or water (depending on how thick you like your shakes) one chopped-up frozen banana, a large scoop of NATURAL peanut butter and a scoop of your favorite chocolate protein powder. Blend on high until desired consistency. You will have to play with the ingredients until you get it down to your liking.

**Dinner-** Pizza! I take a largest wheat/grain tortilla I can find and toast it in the oven until crisp. Rub it with marinara sauce and then cover it with cooked ground turkey breast, mushrooms and a pinch of mozzarella cheese to taste. Flavor with your favorite low-salt Italian or pizza seasoning. If the tortilla is small, have a couple for one serving. Eat until you are full, but not over-the-top! For cheese, watch the salt. Parmigiano-Reggiano and Swiss are naturally lower. Try to stay away from cheese that has more than 400 grams of salt per serving. Lactose intolerant? Try feta as it's naturally lower in lactose. Don't forget to be drinking your target of 8 glasses a day of water!

**Bedtime Snack-** It's a good idea to have a little bit of protein before you go to sleep for the night, you never want to go to bed hungry and protein digests slowly so it's a great choice. I do no more than a cup of light cottage cheese with fruit: a chopped banana or blueberries are delicious with it. Can't do milk products? Have a banana and a large scoop of peanut better.

## Tuesday

**Breakfast-** Heat up multi-grain spinach tortilla and fill it with 3 whole eggs, egg-whites or egg beaters scrambled with a tablespoon of olive oil with spinach. Add a tablespoon of salsa, a pinch of low-fat cheese of your choice. You can sauté the spinach first then add the eggs. Have a glass of water with the meal.

**Mid-Morning Snack-** A handful of chopped strawberries and blueberries glazed with honey. Shave one small piece of bittersweet dark chocolate on top. This makes an amazing desert as well.

**Lunch-** Cold tuna salad. Drain a can of water-packed albacore tuna or a use a dry pack and drop it into your bowl. Mix 1 tablespoon of light mayonnaise, a teaspoon of onion or dill relish and a squeeze a lemon wedge over it. Drop it over your favorite green salad leaves and serve with a banana or your favorite fruit. To make it even easier I just mix in a handful of spinach and roll the mix into a multi-grain tortilla for a balanced and delicious meal.

**Mid-Afternoon Snack-** Brown rice cake with natural peanut butter, sliced banana, glazed with honey. Brown rice cakes are always stocked in my cupboard. They offer a quick, easily packed way to offer me complex carbohydrates. I can put anything on top of them for a nutritionally packed snack. I even have them as a meal if so inclined, I cover them with this same tuna mix- I only end up have 3 or 4 for a meal, just double the tuna.

**Dinner-** Southwestern quinoa and chicken scramble. Take a grilled or broiled chicken breast, dice it and cover it with a cup of heated quinoa and black beans. Cover that with a couple tablespoons of salsa. Add a tablespoon of safflower oil to the salsa, mixed in. If you crave some alcohol, a glass of red wine offers antioxidants so enjoy!

**Nighttime Snack-** A sliced sour-sweet green apple with a scoop of natural peanut butter.

**Bedtime Snack-** Plain Greek yogurt with a portion of your favorite fruit. Berries mixed in the yogurt are my favorite. If you want a little more bulk to this snack, add a couple tablespoons of dry oatmeal or trail mix to it.
You can see how the meals you make can come from pre-prepared basic staple ingredients. It really is easy to make these delicious meals - especially when you have the main ingredients (meat, quinoa, couscous) previously cooked to save time. The next time you are in the house doing other tasks, pre-plan your meals for the week by having these things on hand ready to go. Grill your chicken, turkey, or favorite meat in bulk, freeze it or stick it in the fridge if you. The frozen pieces are great for long drives or flights. Cook up your large servings of quinoa or couscous so you have that, too. Then all you have to do is cover garnish it to your liking and you're in business. It's really that easy!

### _Wednesday_
**Breakfast-** Hot cinnamon couscous cereal with banana and honey. Heat up a cup of pre-cooked couscous, chop up a banana and drop it on top. Sprinkle a light coat of cinnamon on top of that and glaze the top of it all with some honey. Pour a cup of skim or rice milk over it all. Quinoa or steel-cut oats also make great choices.

**Mid-Morning Snack-** 1 cup of fat-free or l% cottage cheese over mixed with cinnamon and raisins. Cottage cheese is one of the best proteins rich in glutamine- this is a muscle preserving amino acid.

**Lunch-** Lemon chicken with a honey-sweet potato. Some of those potatoes are huge so a half, or even a quarter depending upon its size will do. Remember to think of portion sizes, not so much calories. Have the other half for dinner or the next day! It's all about planning ahead. Grilled chicken breast or tenders portion with fresh-squeezed lemon juice and season with garlic powder and crushed black pepper. Micro-wave or previously baked sweet potato, glaze it with honey and a pinch of brown sugar.

**Mid-Afternoon Snack-** Can be as basic as a glass of water with a scoop of your favorite flavored protein powder and fruit. I like to use vanilla or chocolate with rice milk.

**Dinner-** Salmon salad with toasted crushed tortilla crumbs. Broil a salmon steak to desired tenderness (I like to let mine soak in lemon juice overnight) Drop the salmon over a bed of baby spinach leaves, break up toasted multi-grain tortilla over the top. Lightly glaze with your favorite dressing (make your own) Try this one: Mix 2 tablespoons hummus, ½ lemon or lime juice, 1 tablespoon balsamic vinegar and salt and pepper to taste. It makes a delicious dressing that sticks to lettuce leaves very well and compliments any type of meat.
Bedtime snack- 2-3 slices of low-sodium turkey breast meat (found in the deli) on a slice of stone-ground wheat bread. Season lightly with spicy mustard or hummus. The turkey has tryptophan, an amino acid that helps the body make serotonin. Serotonin is a chemical in the brain that aids in the sleep process.

### *Thursday*
**Breakfast-** Apple-flax pancakes. This one is delicious and has a tad more prep time than the other meals I've listed, but the taste and

nutritional values are well worth it. First, the ingredients: 1 egg, 1 Tablespoon plain Greek yogurt, a few drops stevia or agave for sweetening, 1/4 teaspoon vanilla, 2 Tablespoons flax meal (ground flax seeds), 1/3 apple, chopped into 1/4-inch or smaller pieces (you can also use semi-mashed bananas or blueberries.) Beat egg, yogurt and sweetener until mixed thoroughly and fluffy. Stir in flax and fruit, let sit for 2-3 minutes to pre-heat skillet rubbed with coconut oil or sprayed with Pam. Brown on both sides and serve! They are delicious with peanut butter or your favorite fruit preserve spread. Add a large tablespoon of cottage cheese and a glass of water with lemon.

**Mid-Morning Snack-** Fruit medley with ¼ cup dry instant oats, sprinkled with honey

**Lunch-** Out with co-workers! Grilled shrimp tacos with a squeezed lime on yellow corn tortillas, one cup of black beans. No bread appetizers, no soft drinks and no junk! (unless it's your cheat meal) Keep it safe-keep all meats grilled. Sub fries with baked potato, grilled veggies or salad.

**Mid-Afternoon Snack-** Cucumber or zucchini with hummus or celery and peanut butter. A couple pieces will do.

**Dinner-** Grilled chicken tortilla soup. In a small sauce pan, combine one can of chicken broth, a chopped grilled chicken breast, black beans and a handful of your favorite mixed veggies. Frozen will do just fine here, they are just as nutritious as fresh vegetables. Crumble 1-2 corn tortillas on top on the soup and heat for 5 minutes.

**Bedtime Snack-** One banana spread with a tablespoon of peanut butter or your favorite nut butter- the good fat and protein will help you to sleep as well. As a rule, you should not have more than 200 calories for your late-night snack. Digesting full-size meals can sometimes be disruptive if you're trying to fall asleep. Keep it light!

## *Friday*
**Breakfast-** 3 egg whites and ham in a wheat pita sandwich. Scramble the eggs in a small bowl, microwave them on medium for 2-3 minutes. Put in slice of low-sodium ham, sprinkle with low-fat cheddar cheese to taste.

*In the morning, I like to have fruit juice- just keep an eye on the sugar content of these juices. As you know by now, check the labels! I go for grapefruit juice, sweetened by me with stevia or a few drops of lemmon and honey. It's better that way than any company could sweeten it! Another way to limit sugar is to simply dilute the juice, ad half water to your glass.

**Mid-Morning Snack-** Grapefruit sprinkled with honey and a brown rice cake spread with a tablespoon of peanut butter

**Lunch-** Lemmon pepper tuna wraps with spinach. In a bowl mix two cans of tuna, two teaspoons of light mayonnaise and a light a light touch of lemon pepper seasoning. Scoop the tuna into a multi-grain tortilla and cover it with a bed of baby spinach leaves. Makes two wraps. Have with a large glass of water or green tea.

**Mid-Afternoon Snack-** Frozen vanilla protein fruit shake. One scoop of your favorite vanilla protein powder, up to a cup of your favorite low-sugar juice (I use cranberry), 6-8 ice cubes (depending on how thick you like your shakes.) Look for a bag of frozen fruit- various berries or a fruit medley. Grab a large handful an add to your shake, with a tablespoon of flax oil.

**Dinner-** Toasted pita bread stuffed with ground sirloin and vegetables. It's a pita burger! Coat a frying pan with coconut or olive oil and brown the sirloin on medium heat. Add the chopped veggies- a great combo is chopped zucchini, mushroom and onion. Spice to taste, I use garlic powder and cayenne or ground black pepper.

**Bedtime Snack-** One slice of toasted stone ground wheat bread topped with a healthy tablespoon of natural peanut butter and honey. Wash it down with a small glass of skim milk.

There you have them, a whole week of meals that I routinely prepare with various changes in seasoning to mix it up. They are easy, quick and offer the nutrients my body needs to stay in Ultimate shape for the long term. Feel free to mix and match different protein, carbohydrate and vegetable sources from the lists I provided. Don't buy processed foods anymore; period. This alone will have your waistline slimmer and your Abs showing through. After reading this section on nutrition you now know what to look for. When in question, if the item has more than 10 ingredients in it chances are it's unhealthy. Take a minute to always read the labels!

## What about alcohol?

This can be a touchy subject but moderate drinkers appear to maintain better health than abstainers or heavy drinkers- in the long and short term. What is moderation? A maximum of two drinks per day for a man and 1 drink for a woman seems to be the average.

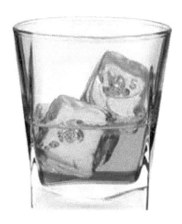

Figure 106: Alcohol

I look at moderate alcohol intake much like consuming healthy fats or exposure to the sun- good for you to a point but can cause problems if you go beyond healthy limits. Even most vitamins our bodies need are toxic if the dosage is too large. Moderate alcohol intake can actually offer some health benefits from lowering high blood pressure, to decreasing hypertension and bouts with the common cold. Just keep it moderate. Go beyond that and you may increase the risk of health problems down the road; indeed there really can be "too much of a good thing".

Some caloric perspective on alcohol vs. other nutrient types:

Fat:  1 gram = 9 calories
Protein: 1 gram = 4 calories
Carbohydrates: 1 gram = 4 calories
Alcohol: 1 gram = 7 calories

An amazing organ, our liver puts all nutrients (good and bad) on the backburner for processing later to dispose of the alcohol first, as it thinks it is toxic. That should explain it- alcohol helps your body store fat and unwanted calories. Ethanol, the type of alcohol found in drinks, has toxic metabolic byproducts called acetaldehyde and acetate. Both by-products help create that queasy nauseous feeling you get when you've thrown too many back. In short, MODERATION. Have a drink, save it as a reward for the weekends. Be a social drinker, never a power drinker. Your fitness, your looks, how you feel, and most importantly your longevity will thank you in the long run.

When it comes to getting in ultimate shape, booze calories can stack up fast if you don't keep track of them. The fact that alcohol contains seven calories per gram and offers zero nutrient content is reason enough to keep it moderate and that's not including all the sugary mixers and additives that some of these drinks include. If you are trying to lose body fat, drinking too much can slow your progress considerably! For starters, how intensely can we train with a hang-over? Alcohol is a diuretic, this is a detriment when the goal is to build and maintain fat-burning muscle. Too much of it causes blood sugar irregularities that shift our hormones to a more "fat-storing" mode than fat-burning one. The take home message here is simple: Keep your alcohol intake consistently minimal if you're going for maximal results!

# CHAPTER 6: The Sessions

Let's now take a look at the final piece to the puzzle- the weight training routines to follow for your specific goal in mind. Notice how I call it weight training and not weight lifting. There is a definite difference. We are doing far more than just moving a weight from point A to point B. For us, the weights and movements are tools to achieve a higher level of health and quality of life- your appearance on the outside may be what you want to improve the most but believe me, what you are going to do for your over-all health, mind and spirit are even more beneficial.

Keep in mind that as you progress, the type of training modes you employ could change as your goals change. This is a normal occurrence and happens often with people that achieve their original goal. For example, an ectomorph that reached his goal of adding 30 pounds of muscle to his frame by consuming enough calories a day and training to gain pure muscle and bodyweight. Now, he takes in less calories and trains with more full-body movements and less rest between sets- different goals require different methods.

We are going to train your body to make the desired changes that you want it to make- through the following scalable modes of training. Are you ready?

## *Training Method for Fat Loss and Inches*

If this is your goal, these workouts are going to center around more constant movement and less rest between sets. We don't always have the free time to train every day - I get that. The beauty of this method is that you don't have to train every day! The key to its success is utilizing supersets of full-body compound movements. This method of weight training works the most important muscle you've got- your heart. It will pump hard and fast- at a cardio pace supplying oxygen-rich blood to all those working muscles. Since all those muscles are working together with minimal rest, it's nearly impossible to use a lot of weight; thus these workouts aren't geared for muscle growth. While still challenging your muscle fibers to "show" more that grow, these workouts are instead geared for extreme heart pumping, fat-stripping results. Use the following guidelines for these supersets:

• Select a weight that allows you to complete reps with moderate difficulty
• Perform each movement within the superset for 12-15 reps in sequence as listed
• Use each sequence for 2-3 weeks then attempt the next level
• Perform the your sprints/cardio any other days out of the week

## Level 1- Two days per week. Example: Monday/Thursday

*Any other days of the week feel free to perform your cardio training

| Superset | Sets | Reps |
|---|---|---|
| 1. Squat-to-shoulder press/ | 3 | 12-15 |
| Modified ball crunch | | |
| Rest 60-120 seconds, perform superset # 2 | | |
| | | |
| 2. Squat-to-bicep curls/Pushups | 3 | 12-15 |
| Rest 60-120 seconds, perform superset # 3 | | |
| | | |
| 3. Bent-over-row/lunge (alternate legs) | 3 | 12-15 |

## Level 2- Three days per week. Example: Monday/Wednesday/Friday

*Select a weight that challenges you to complete reps- pyramid your sets
*Every other day- do you sprint intervals

| Superset | Sets | Reps |
|---|---|---|
| 1. Squat-to-shoulder press/ | 4 | 12-15 |
| Bodyweight row | | |
| Modified ball crunch | | |
| Rest 1 minute, perform superset #2 | | |
| | | |
| 2. Incline dumbbell press/ | 4 | 12-15 |
| Side-step lunge | | |
| Reverse Crunch | | |
| Rest 1 minute, perform superset #3 | | |

| Superset | Sets | Reps |
|---|---|---|
| 3. Lunge-to-upright row/ | 4 | 12-15 |
| Decline push-up | | |
| Rest 1 minute, perform superset #4 | | |

| | | |
|---|---|---|
| 4. Modified swiss ball crunch/ | 4 | 12-15 |
| Bodyweight squat/hanging leg raise | | |

## Level 3- Three days per week. Example: Monday/ Wednesday/Friday

| Superset | Sets | Reps |
|---|---|---|
| 1. Squat-to-shoulder press/ | 4-6 | 12-15 |
| Hanging leg raise (90's) | | |
| Rest 30-45 seconds, perform superset #2 | | |

| | | |
|---|---|---|
| 2. Bent over rows/ | | |
| Flat dumbbell press/ | 4-6 | 12-15 |
| Prone knee-ups | | |
| Rest 30-45 seconds, perform superset #3 | | |

| | | |
|---|---|---|
| 3.Incline dumbbell press/ | 4-6 | 12-15 |
| Swiss ball hand-off | | |
| Rest 10-45 seconds, perform superset #4 | | |

| | | |
|---|---|---|
| 4. Lunge-to-biceps curl/ | 4-6 | 12-15 |
| Decline pushup/ | | |
| Pull-ups | | |

Effective fat burning movements by themselves, these sessions are examples of how to put compound movements together and make supersets that much more effective. Follow them and as you go along mix-and-match movements to keep it interesting- the results will never dissipate the more you mix it up. Stay consistent and never stop moving!

## *Training Method For Weight/Muscle Gain*

The following training method is quite different from the one previously outlined. It is what's called a split schedule, which means focusing on one-two muscle groups per session. It is a more advanced method of training geared toward optimum muscle growth and currently is the type of training I utilize (I use full body and split schedules from time to time) again, mixing it up often. When I say "muscle growth" don't forget that for that to happen more readily you have to be putting in the required amount of calories just as you would have to create a calorie deficit if the goal were to lose weight or inches. As we covered in chapter five, your nutrition and your training work together for the desired results. With this training schedule, each muscle group is trained twice about every eight days- that's three days of rest for each muscle trained, give or take a couple "instinctive" rest days here and there.

The total number of sets for each muscle group is a higher than full-body training sessions, generally no more than 12 for larger muscle groups like back and no more than 8 for smaller groups like arms. The goal here is more muscle growth and with this higher intensity, three days rest is a must for optimum recovery. There are different variations of this method that I employ, each designed to achieve a different goal or evoke a slightly different result. I will list them all for you to follow and use in your own sessions. It does require more days to train with this method but if your goals fit with this method the returns on your efforts are awesome. Let's have a look at a week-long split schedule I use. More specifically, I use a push/pull superset scheme: meaning opposing muscle groups for upper body. Legs have their own day; I usually throw in shoulders with them if I have the energy. As you will see, I still use the superset principle. It simply works that well, keeping up the pace and saving me time. I can get in and out of the gym in about 45 minutes and still get a killer session.

## Guidelines for the split schedule

- Use high intensity- pyramid your sets and challenge yourself
- Keep rest between sets minimal- no more than 90 seconds
- Always start with a compound movement- last movements can be isolation
- Every workout should be different- change angles and movements often

*This particular schedule is a push/pull superset. Meaning, the chest is a pushing muscle group and the biceps are a pulling muscle. They are opposing muscle groups and as such, allow you to put more effort into each set because you are not using either one to help the other during the set such as triceps helping chest push the barbell up. This allows you to conserve more energy for each targeted muscle group. More intensity means faster results!

- Perform a minimum of two movements per muscle group, no more than four
- I work calves in every 2-3 days, usually at the end of my session

- I work Abs every 2-3 days, pairing them with different muscle groups/days. Pick movements to superset. Example: hanging leg raise/stability ball crunch- 4 supersets
- Days off- I take two days "instinctively" when I don't feel like training that day
- I run hill sprints generally on upper body days or days off-instinctive as well

## Monday- Chest/Biceps

| Exercise | Super Sets |
|---|---|
| Smith Incline press/Seat incline dumbbell curls | 4 |
| Flat dumbbell press/Standing barbell curls | 4 |
| Cable-cross overs/seated concentration curls | 3 |
| Calves- seated calf raises/standing bodyweight raises (on a block) | 4 |

## Tuesday- Legs/Abs

| | |
|---|---|
| Dumbbell squat/Swiss ball crunch | 4 |
| Smith Lunge/incline reverse crunch | 4 |
| Stiff-legged dead lifts/hanging leg raise | 4 |

## Wednesday- Day Off/Hillsprints          30 minutes

## Thursday- Back/Shoulders/Triceps

| | |
|---|---|
| Seated dumbbell shoulder press/lat pulls | 4 |
| Bent-over rows/lying triceps extension | 4 |
| Lateral raises/triceps pushdown | 4 |
| Calves- Leg press (swapped for standing raise)/ seated raise | 4 |

## Friday-Chest Biceps (repeat cycle just different movements)

| | |
|---|---|
| Incline dumbbell press/Seated hammer curls | 4 |
| Flat smith press/bodyweight curls | 4 |
| Peck-deck | 3 |

## Saturday- Legs/Abs

| | |
|---|---|
| Leg press/bodyweight lunges | 5 |
| Swiss ball hamstring curls/side bridges | 4 |
| Hanging leg raises (non-90's- easier!) | 4 |

## Sunday- day off from weights/hills prints    30 minutes

## Monday- Back/Shoulders/Triceps

| Exercise | Super Sets |
|---|---|
| Pull-ups/Upright rows (bar) | 5 |
| Bent-over rows (bar) overhead tricep extension | 5 |
| Front/lateral raises/reverse grip pushdowns | 4 |
| Calves- Leg press (swapped for standing raise)/seated raise | |

## Tuesday- Chest/Biceps

| | |
|---|---|
| Bench press/dumbbell curls | 5 |
| Incline flys/reverse grip barbell curls | 5 |
| Low cable flys | 4 |

## Wednesday – Day Off/Hillsprints    30 minutes

## Thursday- Legs/Abs

| | |
|---|---|
| Modified-smith lunges/bodyweight squats | 5 |
| Stiff-legged dead lifts/side lunges | 5 |
| Roll-outs/seated leg-raises | 3 |
| Swill ball crunch/circle leg lifts | 3 |

Again, this is the method I employ mainly because my body type being historically ectomorphic responds very well to this type of training, my goals are achieved as a result and yours will be too. The main points of this or any type of schedule are simple: Train and eat for your body type and goals. Be consistent, intense and always use Great Form down to every single workout, set and rep!

# In Closing

Things will inevitably be challenging. Some days you won't even want to look at a weight much less try to lift one. I certainly have those days. It's okay! This is what off-days and cheat days are for. Use them wisely and use them for days like these. Your diet won't always be on point either. Just make the effort to be consistent. Reward yourself often with a cheat meal here and there within reason. When you are consistent in your methods week after week, month after month, your body will be given no choice but to improve- don't give it any slack. Leave yourself no choice but success. Thank you for allowing me to help coach and motivate you toward your fitness goals. As a fitness professional it is my job to coach clients in the most effective and safe methods for ultimate results. I feel the most successful trainers teach their clients to a point but in the long run provide enough knowledge and motivation for the client to develop and coach themselves for constant improvement.

To quote the late Bruce Lee- "I am not teaching you anything, I just help you to explore yourself." With the right tools, the sky is the limit and you are in control. Get the body and life you want, and start getting it NOW. Your Ultimate Body! Those Awesome Abs are sure to follow!

See you in the gym!